Healthy Technology Use

Healthy Technology Use

Your Questions Answered

Bernadette H. Schell

BLOOMSBURY ACADEMIC
NEW YORK • LONDON • OXFORD • NEW DELHI • SYDNEY

BLOOMSBURY ACADEMIC
Bloomsbury Publishing Inc
1385 Broadway, New York, NY 10018, USA
50 Bedford Square, London, WC1B 3DP, UK
29 Earlsfort Terrace, Dublin 2, Ireland

BLOOMSBURY, BLOOMSBURY ACADEMIC and the Diana logo
are trademarks of Bloomsbury Publishing Plc

First published in the United States of America 2024

Library of Congress Cataloging-in-Publication Data
Names: Schell, Bernadette H. (Bernadette Hlubik), 1952- author.
Title: Healthy technology use : your questions answered / Bernadette H. Schell.
Description: New York : Bloomsbury Academic, 2024. |
Series: Q&A health guides | Includes index. | Audience: Grades 10–12
Identifiers: LCCN 2023058266 (print) | LCCN 2023058267 (ebook) |
ISBN 9781440880605 (HB) | ISBN 9781440880612 (ePDF) | ISBN 9798765110379 (eBook)
Subjects: LCSH: Technology–Miscellanea–Juvenile literature. | Technology–Health
aspects–Juvenile literature. | Technology–Psychological aspects–Juvenile literature. |
Technological innovations–Psychological aspects–Juvenile literature. |
Information technology–Psychological aspects–Juvenile literature.
Classification: LCC T48 .S4147 2024 (print) | LCC T48 (ebook) |
DDC 303.48/3–dc23/eng/20240227
LC record available at https://lccn.loc.gov/2023058266
LC ebook record available at https://lccn.loc.gov/2023058267

ISBN: HB: 978-1-4408-8060-5
         ePDF: 978-1-4408-8061-2
         eBook: 979-8-7651-1037-9

Series: Q&A Health Guides

Typeset by Integra Software Services Pvt. Ltd.
Printed and bound in the United States of America

To find out more about our authors and books visit www.bloomsbury.com
and sign up for our newsletters.

Contents

Contents

Case Studies

Series Foreword

All of us have questions about our health. Is this normal? Should I be doing something differently? Whom should I talk to about my concerns? And our modern world is full of answers. Thanks to the internet, there's a wealth of information at our fingertips, from forums where people can share their personal experiences to Wikipedia articles to the full text of medical studies. But finding the right information can be an intimidating and difficult task—some sources are written at too high a level, others have been oversimplified, while still others are heavily biased or simply inaccurate.

Q&A Health Guides address the needs of readers who want accurate, concise answers to their health questions, authored by reputable and objective experts, and written in clear and easy-to-understand language. This series focuses on the topics that matter most to young adult readers, including various aspects of physical and emotional well being as well as other components of a healthy lifestyle. These guides will also serve as a valuable tool for parents, school counselors, and others who may need to answer teens' health questions.

All books in the series follow the same format to make finding information quick and easy. Each volume begins with an essay on health literacy and why it is so important when it comes to gathering and evaluating health information. Next, the top five myths and misconceptions that surround the topic are dispelled. The heart of each guide is a collection of questions and answers, organized thematically. A selection of five case studies provides real-world examples to illuminate key concepts. Rounding out each volume are a directory of resources, glossary, and index. It is our hope that the books in this series will not only provide valuable information but will also help guide readers toward a lifetime of healthy decision-making.

Acknowledgments

Many thanks to Maxine Taylor, who—as always—assisted me greatly in bringing this project to fruition.

Introduction

As a former stress management industry consultant and a long-time professor of Business and Information Technology in Canada, I found in earlier days that students would often ask me questions like, "How can I best make lots of money and also benefit society with my new business idea?" But in recent I have found a shift in our conversations from a focus on how best to capitalize on business and social investment returns to a more self-focused angle. For example, students are searching for practical answers to questions like, "How can I maintain my own work-life balance while being actively engaged in a fast-paced, high-tech work or study environment?"

I often respond with these four simple words, "Through healthy technology use." Pragmatic conversations are typically then generated by students around the many facets of healthy technology use. They share comments like "I'd like to hear more about how I can safeguard myself from mental, physical, or financial harms—or bad actors—while working or studying, or relating to my friends online." Or they ask probing questions, such as "How do I know if I am over-using my digital devices, or even becoming addicted to them?"

Topics like these have informed the outline on which this healthy technology use book was based. This book's purpose is to provide you with experts' practical recommendations on important personal online safety information, such as these:

- *Understanding the negative impact of technology over-use on your mental health, relationships, and achievement.* For example, how do you know if you are using social media excessively or playing online games too much? And if you think that you may have a problem in this regard, how do you know if you need professional help to effectively deal with your issue?
- *Understanding the negative impact of technology over-use on your physical health and safety.* For example, how does over-using technology negatively affect your sleep? Or, to help keep you safe while online, what user protection features are built into social media and messaging apps?
- *Understanding how to safeguard your money and your identity while online.* For example, what should you do if you believe you are the victim of

online fraud? Or, how can you protect yourself from becoming a victim of online identity theft?

- *Understanding how going online can affect your privacy, make you a party to piracy, or bombard you with fake news or harmful disinformation.* For example, why do online social media companies collect so much of your personal information, and what do they do with it? What should you do if you are receiving unwanted sexts from someone after using social media? Can you freely share with your friends some movies or songs you downloaded for your own use—without violating copyright laws?
- *Addressing technology over-use with real-world, practical solutions.* For example, what does "being mindful about technology use" really mean? Or if your friends sometimes talk about doing a "digital detox," what exactly is one, and what are the costs and benefits for you?

This book also discusses five common misconceptions about healthy technology use, clarifying fact from fiction. For example, if you've heard that antisocial teens are the only people negatively affected by the over-use of technology, how true is this? Or, if you've heard friends say that doing a "digital detox" is only beneficial for people who are truly addicted to the internet or social media, how true is this?

This book also shares five interesting case examples of people questioning their own healthy technology use. It offers some practical ways that these individuals can maintain their financial or mental well-being—or recover from the psychological or physical harms resulting from overexposure to it. It closes with a glossary of terms and a directory of resources that may be helpful to you to better understand this topic.

I hope that this book enlightens you about how to develop an effective regimen around healthy technology use—and offers some useful pointers on when to seek professional help if you think you are not doing as well as you should at safeguarding your well being and keeping yourself safe while online.

Guide to Health Literacy

On her thirteenth birthday, Samantha was diagnosed with type 2 diabetes. She consulted her mom and her aunt, both of whom also have type 2 diabetes, and decided to go with their strategy of managing diabetes by taking insulin. As a result of participating in an after-school program at her middle school that focused on health literacy, she learned that she can help manage the level of glucose in her bloodstream by counting her carbohydrate intake, following a diabetic diet, and exercising regularly. But, what exactly should she do? How does she keep track of her carbohydrate intake? What is a diabetic diet? How long should she exercise and what type of exercise should she do? Samantha is a visual learner, so she turned to her favorite source of media, YouTube, to answer these questions. She found videos from individuals around the world sharing their experiences and tips, doctors (or at least people who have "Dr." in their YouTube channel names), government agencies such as the National Institutes of Health, and even video clips from cat lovers who have cats with diabetes. With guidance from the librarian and the health and science teachers at her school, she assessed the credibility of the information in these videos and even compared their suggestions to some of the print resources that she was able to find at her school library. Now, she knows exactly how to count her carbohydrate level, how to prepare and follow a diabetic diet, and how much (and what) exercise is needed daily. She intends to share her findings with her mom and her aunt, and now she wants to create a chart that summarizes what she has learned that she can share with her doctor.

Samantha's experience is not unique. She represents a shift in our society; an individual no longer views himself or herself as a passive recipient of medical care but as an active mediator of his or her own health. However, in this era when any individual can post his or her opinions and experiences with a particular health condition online with just a few clicks or publish a memoir, it is vital that people know how to assess the credibility of health information. Gone are the days when "publishing" health information required intense vetting. The health information landscape is highly saturated, and people have innumerable sources where they can find information about practically any health topic. The sources (whether print, online, or a person) that an individual consults for health information are crucial because the accuracy and trustworthiness of the information can potentially affect his or her overall health. The ability to find, select, assess, and use health information constitutes a type of literacy—health literacy—that everyone must possess.

The Definition and Phases of Health Literacy

One of the most popular definitions for health literacy comes from Ratzan and Parker (2000), who describe health literacy as "the degree to which individuals have the capacity to obtain, process, and understand basic health information and services needed to make appropriate health decisions." Recent research has extrapolated health literacy into health literacy bits, further shedding light on the multiple phases and literacy practices that are embedded within the multifaceted concept of health literacy. Although this research has focused primarily on online health information seeking, these health literacy bits are needed to successfully navigate both print and online sources. There are six phases of health information seeking: (1) Information Need Identification and Question Formulation, (2) Information Search, (3) Information Comprehension, (4) Information Assessment, (5) Information Management, and (6) Information Use.

The first phase is the *information need identification and question formulation phase.* In this phase, one needs to be able to develop and refine a range of questions to frame one's search and understand relevant health terms. In the second phase, *information search,* one has to possess appropriate searching skills, such as using proper keywords and correct spelling in search terms, especially when using search engines and databases. It is also crucial to understand how search engines work (i.e., how search results are derived, what the order of the search results means, how to use the snippets that are provided in the search results list to select websites, and how to determine which listings are ads on a search engine results page). One also has to limit reliance on surface characteristics, such as the design of a website or a book (a website or book that appears to have a lot of information or looks aesthetically pleasant does not necessarily mean it has good information) and language used (a website or book that utilizes jargon, the keywords that one used to conduct the search, or the word "information" does not necessarily indicate it will have good information). The next phase is *information comprehension,* whereby one needs to have the ability to read, comprehend, and recall the information (including textual, numerical, and visual content) one has located from the books and/or online resources.

To assess the credibility of health information (*information assessment phase*), one needs to be able to evaluate information for accuracy, evaluate how current the information is (e.g., when a website was last updated or when a book was published), and evaluate the creators of the source—for example, examine site sponsors or type of sites (.com, .gov, .edu, or .org) or the author of a book (practicing doctor, a celebrity doctor, a patient of a specific disease, etc.) to determine the believability of the person/organization providing the information. Such credibility perceptions tend to become generalized, so they must be frequently reexamined (e.g., the belief that a specific news agency always has credible health information needs continuous vetting). One also needs to evaluate the credibility of the medium (e.g., television, internet, radio, social media, and book) and evaluate—not just accept without questioning—others' claims regarding the validity of a site, book, or other specific source of information. At this stage, one has to "make sense of information gathered from diverse sources by identifying misconceptions, main and supporting ideas, conflicting information, point of view, and biases" (American Association of School Librarians [AASL], 2009, p. 13) and conclude which sources/information are valid and accurate by using conscious strategies rather than simply using intuitive judgments or "rules of thumb." This phase is the most challenging segment of health information-seeking and serves as a determinant of success (or lack thereof) in the information-seeking process. The following section on Sources of Health Information further explains this phase.

The fifth phase is *information management*, whereby one has to organize information that has been gathered in some manner to ensure easy retrieval and use in the future. The last phase is *information use*, in which one will synthesize information found across various resources, draw conclusions, and locate the answer to his or her original question and/or the content that fulfills the information need. This phase also often involves implementation, such as using the information to solve a health problem; make health-related decisions; identify and engage in behaviors that will help a person avoid health risks; share the health information found with family members and friends who may benefit from it; and advocate more broadly for personal, family, or community health.

The Importance of Health Literacy

The conception of health has moved from a passive view (someone is either well or ill) to one that is more active and process based (someone is working toward preventing or managing disease). Hence, the dominant focus has shifted from doctors and treatments to patients and prevention, resulting in the need to strengthen our ability and confidence (as patients and consumers of health care) to look for, assess, understand, manage, share, adapt, and use health-related information. An individual's health literacy level has been found to predict his or her health status better than age, race, educational attainment, employment status, and income level (National Network of Libraries of Medicine, 2013). Greater health literacy also enables individuals to better communicate with health care providers such as doctors, nutritionists, and therapists, as they can pose more relevant, informed, and useful questions to health care providers. Another added advantage of greater health literacy is better information-seeking skills, not only for health but also in other domains, such as completing assignments for school.

Sources of Health Information: The Good, the Bad, and the In-Between

For generations, doctors, nurses, nutritionists, health coaches, and other health professionals have been the trusted sources of health information. Additionally, researchers have found that young adults, when they have health-related questions, typically turn to a family member who has had firsthand experience with a health condition because of their family member's close proximity and because of their past experience with, and trust in, this individual. Expertise should be a core consideration when consulting a person, website, or book for health information. The credentials and background of the person or author and conflicting interests of the author (and his or her organization) must be checked and validated to ensure the likely credibility of the health information they are conveying. While books often have implied credibility because of the peer-review process involved, self-publishing has challenged this credibility, so qualifications of book authors should also be verified. When it comes to health information, currency of the source must also be examined. When examining health information/studies presented, pay attention to the exhaustiveness of research methods utilized to offer recommendations or conclusions. Small and non-diverse sample size is often—but not always—an indication of reduced credibility. Studies that confuse correlation with causation is another potential issue to watch for. Information seekers must also pay attention to the sponsors of the research studies. For example, if a study is sponsored by manufacturers of drug Y and the study recommends that drug Y is the best treatment to manage or cure a disease, this may indicate a lack of objectivity on the part of the researchers.

The internet is rapidly becoming one of the main sources of health information. Online forums, news agencies, personal blogs, social media sites, pharmacy sites, and celebrity "doctors" are all offering medical and health information targeted to various types of people in regard to all types of diseases and symptoms. There are professional journalists, citizen journalists, hoaxers, and people paid to write fake health news on various sites that may appear to have a legitimate domain name and may even have authors who claim to have professional credentials, such as an MD. All these sites *may* offer useful information or information that appears to be useful and relevant; however, much of the information may be debatable and may fall into gray areas that require readers to discern credibility, reliability, and biases.

While broad recognition and acceptance of certain media, institutions, and people often serve as the most popular determining factors to assess credibility of health information among young people, keep in mind that there are legitimate internet sites, databases, and books that publish health information and serve as sources of health information for doctors, other health sites, and members of the public. For example, MedlinePlus (https://medlineplus.gov) has trusted sources on over 975 diseases and conditions and presents the information in easy-to-understand language.

The chart here presents factors to consider when assessing credibility of health information. However, keep in mind that these factors function only as a guide and require continuous updating to keep abreast with the changes in the landscape of health information, information sources, and technologies.

The chart can serve as a guide; however, approaching a librarian about how one can go about assessing the credibility of both print and online health information is far more effective than using generic checklist-type tools. While librarians are not health experts, they can apply and teach patrons strategies to determine the credibility of health information.

With the prevalence of fake sites and fake resources that appear to be legitimate, it is important to use the following health information assessment tips to verify health information that one has obtained (St. Jean et al., 2015, p. 151):

- **Don't assume you are right**: Even when you feel very sure about an answer, keep in mind that the answer may not be correct, and it is important to conduct (further) searches to validate the information.

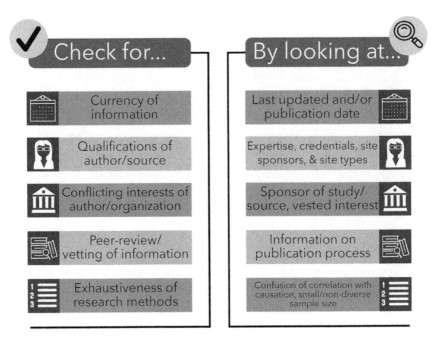

All images from flaticon.com

- **Don't assume you are wrong**: You may actually have correct information, even if the information you encounter does not match—that is, you may be right and the resources that you have found may contain false information.
- **Take an open approach**: Maintain a critical stance by not including your preexisting beliefs as keywords (or letting them influence your choice of keywords) in a search, as this may influence what it is possible to find out.
- **Verify, verify, and verify**: Information found, especially on the internet, needs to be validated, no matter how the information appears on the site (i.e., regardless of the appearance of the site or the quantity of information that is included).

Health literacy comes with experience navigating health information. Professional sources of health information, such as doctors, health care providers, and health databases, are still the best, but one also has the power to search for health information and then verify it by consulting with these trusted sources and by using the health information assessment tips and guide shared previously.

Mega Subramaniam, Ph.D.
Associate Professor, College of Information Studies,
University of Maryland

References and Further Reading

American Association of School Librarians (AASL) (2009). *Standards for the 21st-century learner in action.* Chicago, IL: American Association of School Librarians.

Hilligoss, B., & Rieh, S.-Y. (2008). Developing a unifying framework of credibility assessment: Construct, heuristics, and interaction in context. *Information Processing & Management,* 44(4), 1467–84.

Kuhlthau, C. C. (1988). Developing a model of the library search process: Cognitive and affective aspects. *Reference Quarterly,* 28(2), 232–42.

National Network of Libraries of Medicine (NNLM) (2013). *Health literacy.* Bethesda, MD: National Network of Libraries of Medicine. Retrieved from nnlm.gov/outreach/consumer/hlthlit.html

Ratzan, S. C., & Parker, R. M. (2000). Introduction. In C. R. Selden, M. Zorn, S. C. Ratzan, & R. M. Parker (Eds.), *National Library of Medicine current bibliographies in medicine: Health literacy.* NLM Pub. No. CBM 2000–1. Bethesda, MD: National Institutes of Health, U.S. Department of Health and Human Services.

St. Jean, B., Subramaniam, M., Taylor, N. G., Follman, R., Kodama, C., & Casciotti, D. (2015). The influence of positive hypothesis testing on youths' online health-related information seeking. *New Library World,* 116(3/4), 136–54.

St. Jean, B., Taylor, N. G., Kodama, C., & Subramaniam, M. (February 2017). Assessing the health information source perceptions of tweens using card-sorting exercises. *Journal of Information Science.* Retrieved from http://journals.sagepub.com/doi/abs/10.1177/0165551516687728

Subramaniam, M., St. Jean, B., Taylor, N. G., Kodama, C., Follman, R., & Casciotti, D. (2015). Bit by bit: Using design-based research to improve the health literacy of adolescents. *JMIR Research Protocols,* 4(2), paper e62. Retrieved from http://www.ncbi.nlm.nih.gov/pmc/articles/PMC4464334/

Valenza, J. (November 26, 2016). *Truth, truthiness, and triangulation: A news literacy toolkit for a "post-truth" world* [Web log]. Retrieved from http://blogs.slj.com/neverendingsearch/2016/11/26/truth-truthiness-triangulation-and-the-librarian-way-a-news-literacy-toolkit-for-a-post-truth-world/

Common Misconceptions about Healthy Technology Use

1. Antisocial teens are the only people negatively affected by the over-use of technology

You may think that only antisocial teens who prefer to communicate with peers primarily through their computers rather than face-to-face are the only ones prone to over-using technology. But think again. The reality is that all individuals who rely on technology to enjoy life are capable of over-using it and even becoming addicted to it. In fact, the general notion of internet addiction was first talked about in 1995 when psychologist Dr. Kimberly Young discussed its worrisome prevalence among online users in the United States. Since then, researchers across a number of disciplines globally have documented the many negative effects associated with technology over-use in the general population—and not just in anti-social teens. This disorder has been linked to a variety of mental, physical, relationship, and productivity health issues, including experiencing high levels of anxiety, depression, and stress. The recent multiple lockdowns because of the Covid-19 pandemic shed light on this truth. At that time, people of all ages required a daily online lifeline for work or school, and some became concerned about their own symptoms of technology over-use. Unfortunately, many teens who already had a problem with digital device over-use in so-called "normal" times were assessed by mental health experts to be particularly vulnerable to increased mental and physical harms during the lockdowns. For more detailed information about when you should seek professional help for digital device over-use or internet addiction, see questions 2 and 3.

2. Firewalls and antivirus software are effective at keeping your computer and information safe

While a good firewall and a reliable virus scanner are crucial to protect computers and the information contained in them, many users *falsely* believe that this two-pronged safety approach will *totally* stop bad actors from invading and doing harm. Not so. By definition, a firewall is a security mechanism protecting unauthorized access by bad actors by monitoring incoming and outgoing internet traffic on the network. It decides which requests (data packets) go in and out (i.e., are "safe") based on a set of security "rules" or protocols. The precise rules a firewall applies to determine "clean" traffic vary widely. But firewalls are not 100 percent foolproof! Sometimes a firewall is not properly configured and is unable to prevent all threats because the rules are not strict enough, or it malfunctions because updates are overdue. Also, there could be hardware-related limitations. Malicious files can then find their way onto users' computers through a spam link, a file download, or a flash drive. So, extra help is needed. Antivirus software provides another layer of protection by scanning, spotting, and obliterating or segregating the corrupt files (i.e., malware) that have evaded detection. But like firewalls, commercial anti-virus software products (like *McAfee* or *F-secure*) are not 100 percent foolproof! For years, creative virus writers have been using code-morphing techniques to avoid detection by altering the machine code of the virus program, while maintaining its malicious functionality. Thus, the virus "fingerprint" is changed—and detection by anti-virus software is cleverly avoided. The bottom line is this: Online users need to not only install *both* a good firewall and antivirus software but *must keep both current* to avert as many dangers as possible. For more detailed information about how you can protect your system against particular kinds of malware like phishing, spam, and ransomware, see questions 24 and 28.

3. The safety features built into social networking websites protect users from cyberbullying and cyberharassment

If you think that Social Networking Sites (SNSs) like *Facebook* and *Twitter* (now *X*) have built-in features to keep you safe from cyber bullies and cyber harassers when you connect online, consider these facts. Experts in a number of fields—including mental health, cyber security, criminology, and business—allege that SNSs not only lack built-in design features to keep users safe but can expose you to serious online abuses. Mental health experts have also warned that spending excessive time on SNSs can rob you of precious sleep, zap your concentration and achievement at school or work, cause you real-world relationship deterioration issues, and erode your self-esteem and mental health. A global media-covered case of online abuse resulting in a young person's suicide occurred in 2012. It was that of fifteen-year-old Canadian Amanda Todd, who was cyber bullied, cyber

xxii   *Common Misconceptions about Healthy Technology Use*

stalked, and cyber extorted in *Facebook* for two years by a Dutch man found guilty of serially abusing adolescents online in the Netherlands and elsewhere. So what makes SNSs so perilous? Whistleblower Frances Haugen, a former data scientist at *Facebook*, testified before a US Senate subcommittee in 2021 that not only SNSs sow division and undermine democracy through their pursuit of huge profits gained through controversy and targeted ads toward users, but they choose to maximize wealth over designing and implementing safeguards for platform users. She said that *Facebook* intentionally hid from the public and government officials their own internal research illustrating the harms of its products on users. Haugen urged lawmakers to examine the algorithms (i.e., formulas) driving popular features—such as the main feeds in *Facebook*—where user engagement is rewarded through platform design features such as "Likes." She argued that user engagement algorithms advance all forms of sensational content (and company profits)—including posts featuring rage, hate toward designated groups, or misinformation. Soon after this *Facebook* revelation, a similar expose erupted in 2022 for *Twitter*. For more details on how you can guard against harms while on SNSs, see questions 16, 18, 20, and 33.

4. Doing a "digital detox" is only beneficial for people who are truly addicted to the internet

Are some of your friends talking about doing a "digital detox" when you thought that those were only useful for users addicted to the internet? A "digital detox" is when an internet user intentionally switches off all mobiles, tablets, smartphones, laptops, and computers for a certain length of time to reduce his or her stress levels, focusing on land-based social interactions rather connecting with friends primarily in the virtual world. Though the science of how technology over-use negatively affects our well-being is still in its infancy, the concept of doing a "digital detox" to maintain health is not a new idea. It actually appeared in the *Oxford Dictionary* in 2013. In fact, psychologist Dr. Kimberley Young publicly stated in 1996 that almost 20 percent of college-aged users in the United States suffered from "Internet addiction"—and that maybe they should consider taking a break from internet connectivity to become more mentally and physically balanced. With the proliferation of enticing digital devices on the market, Dr. Young later affirmed that the percentage of young adult internet and digital device "addicts" continues to spiral annually. She also said that once a young adult becomes digitally addicted, he or she has to be ready to complete a "digital detox" before any kind of mental health therapy will have any chance of being effective. Therefore, she urged *all* young adults to routinely practice taking a break from technology to maintain their mental and physical well-being and to lower their risk of becoming a so-called "digital junkie." In short, doing a "digital detox" is beneficial for anyone, not just for those professionally assessed as being clinically addicted. For additional useful information to determine if you are using the internet, social media, or online games in excess—and when you should seek professional help to deal with your concerns, see questions 2, 3, 4, 6, 16, 44, 49, and 52.

5. The only way to effectively fight technology over-use is to go "cold turkey" and stop using devices altogether

In a Deloitte 2017 UK study, when young adults in the 16–24 age category were asked how best to reduce their excessive smartphone usage, the majority said that they should "remove the temptation altogether." But does this finding suggest to you that effectively fighting technology over-use means going "cold turkey"? The good news is that over the past decade, a number of mediating alternatives have been created, tested, and recommended by mental health experts. While most of these do require some form of digital detox at the start, the goal of the mediating alternatives is to gradually have users introduce a healthier digital device regimen into their lives. Some of these options come with a heftier price tag for implementation, so many device over-users prefer starting with the less costly remedies to assess their effectiveness before moving on to the more costly and time-consuming ones. At the lower cost end are reading books offering "digital disconnect" advice, doing a weekly religious-based Shabbat, installing special apps on your smartphone to mindfully limit its use, joining a fellowship group such as The internet and Tech Addicts Anonymous (ITAA), or attending free classes at school or in the community specially designed to help break the digital device over-use cycle. At the pricier end are suggestions such as attending special "digital detox" weekend camps like Camp Grounded, visiting designated digital detox resorts alone or with family members, or registering for therapy sessions with a mental health expert specially trained in internet addiction and digital device rehabilitation. For additional information on the various options available to you to moderate your internet and digital device usage, see questions 44, 46, 47, 48, 49, 51, 52, 53, and 54.

Questions and Answers

The Negative Impact of Technology Over-Use on Mental Health, Relationships, and Achievement

1. Is the internet addictive?

Have you ever wondered if the internet is addictive? The reality is that any kind of activity you intensely and routinely engage in can eventually become an "addiction" if that behavior becomes a dysfunctional obsession of yours. From a historical angle, the notion of internet addiction has been around since the 1970s when elite computer programmers and good guy computer hackers were often referred to as "computer addicts." They were not viewed negatively but as really smart people who sat in front of their computers for twenty or more hours at one time to be positive contributors to technology development and society. Then in the 1990s, things started to change. The high-profile US case of the late hacker Kevin Mitnick, imprisoned for years because of the damages he purportedly caused by his obsessive hacking exploits, helped legitimize the notion of "clinical computer addiction" in the field of mental health.

In fact, it was in 1995 that the term "Internet Addiction Disorder," or IAD, was coined by US psychiatrist Dr. Ivan Goldberg to describe pathological and obsessive computer use among even mainstream digital users, not just hackers. Interestingly, he actually first used the term as a joke to describe his own intense, routine use of the internet when communicating with fellow psychiatrists. But in 1996, Dr. Goldberg more seriously suggested that the clinical or diagnostic criteria for IAD would not be much different from those assigned to Substance Abuse Disorder (aka SAD)—but involve obsessive computer use instead of substance use. He argued that folks impacted by IAD would experience reduced well-being because of their debilitating symptoms related to internet tolerance and withdrawal—thereby forgoing or reducing important social, school, or occupational activities previously enjoyed in the land-based world to "be present" in the virtual world. Though he estimated that the global prevalence of internet addiction in the 1990s likely ranged from 6 percent to 38 percent in the general population, the question remains to this day: Is the internet itself addictive?

While some mental health experts believe that the term *addiction* should be strictly reserved for cases involving substance abuse and not computers or the internet, a growing majority believe the internet is addictive—leading to many types of online obsessions—including Social Networking Site (SNS) addiction, Internet Gaming Disorder (IGD), smartphone addiction, news-watching addiction, and binge-watching addiction. In 2014, Professor Mark Griffiths of Nottingham Trent University in the UK and his colleague Attila Szabo suggested that *both* internet activities and the internet itself are addictive sources. It seems reasonable, they said, that concepts like SNS addiction and smartphone addiction can be considered to be real, harmful, present-day problems in which the "addicting substance" is the internet. While the debate continues and the verdict is still out on whether the internet is itself addictive, US mental health expert Dr. Kimberly Young cautioned in 2016 that society cannot ignore that there is a problem with over-use of the internet in all of its forms.

2. How do you know if you are using the internet, social media, or online games too much? How do you know if you need professional help to deal with this problem?

If you think that you might be seriously overdoing it by constantly connecting to social SNSs or playing online games—to the point that you're pondering whether you should see a professional for assessment, we will now explore some helpful pointers advanced by mental health experts to help you decide what to do next.

For starters, in the mental health community, an addiction is broadly defined as some compulsive, continued use of a substance (like alcohol or drugs) *or* a repeated behavior (as in playing online games for hours or days without taking a break). Users who take part in these behaviors over some length of time tend to experience physical and/or emotional harms. In this context, an addiction is often described by experts in psychology and criminology as being symptomatic of an Impulse Control Disorder (ICD)—essentially, being unable to stop engaging in the troubling behavior or using the troubling substance.

Now let's take a closer look at what ICD means in terms of social media over-use. Suppose you know that overdoing it on social media will eventually have some negative consequences for you, but you keep connecting anyway to gratify your desire (or impulse) to constantly communicate with friends, day and night. Experts say that you will know you have crossed the invisible safety line when you routinely fail to get enough sleep at night, or you find yourself unable to achieve at school the next day because you are tired and you didn't prepare for assignments.

In 1996, Dr. Kimberly Young, a psychology professor at the University of Pittsburgh (and later Dr. Gerald Block in 2008) said that in teens counselled for online addiction, they often experienced a number of negative behaviors. For example, they: (1) found themselves withdrawing from daily activities they previously enjoyed; (2) had tolerance issues, such as needing to buy a better smartphone with more "connect" features so they could spend more "quality" time in social media; (3) were preoccupied with the "behavior of concern," such that they couldn't stop thinking about, say, connecting to their favorite social media site; (4) centralized their other daily activities to procure more time to engage in social media—often experiencing anger, tension, and/or depression when they couldn't connect; (5) lost interest in other social, school, work, or recreational activities they formerly enjoyed; and (6) denied there was a deterioration in their well-being—including the physical, psychological, achievement, and relationship aspects.

If you find that these traits pretty well describe your behavior in terms of internet, social media, or gaming over-use, you may want to complete one of the free self-report inventories developed by mental health experts to help you determine if you are at risk for internet addiction. Alternatively, you can make an appointment with a mental health professional, who will likely ask you to complete some validated inventories. You would receive feedback from the expert about whether you are at low, moderate, or high risk for addiction, based on your answers.

To give you an idea of what you can expect, one such popular twenty-item inventory known as the Short Form of the Internet Addiction Test (s-IAT) was developed by Dr. Young and colleagues and is available on her treatment center's NetAddiction website.

3. What are the different kinds of internet over-use, and are some more concerning than others?

Yearly, it seems as though new kinds of so-called internet addiction types appear in the media. But, according to mental health experts, some of these are more concerning than others because of the reported harms experienced by users. These types are wide-ranging and have included email-checking, news-checking, binge-watching, social networking, and online gaming. Let's now look at how these types are defined, what users' behavior patterns typically look like, what motivates users to engage in these behaviors, and known harms affecting online over-users or addicts.

Let's start with email addiction—a phenomenon that the media discuss quite often but to which mental health experts have given relatively little air time. As far as we know, this type surfaced in 2006 when Dr. Tom Stafford, a UK psychologist at the University of Sheffield, referred to it in a blog post on *Mind Hacks*. He said he was worried about his own compulsion to hit the "get mail" button at least a hundred times a day, and if he didn't get any new mail, he confessed, he would hit the button again! Dr. Stafford knew that he likely wouldn't find anything interesting, that he should concentrate on his work instead, and that as a psych professor, he should know better than to engage in this obsessive behavior pattern.

Why then did Dr. Stafford engage in this behavior? The key, he said, is operant conditioning—the way that humans' and animals' behavior is shaped by results from the perceived consequences occurring following the behavior. Simply put, if you perceive a behavior to be rewarding, you would repeat it. But if you perceive it to be punishing, you would avoid it, and the behavior would eventually be extinguished. Dr. Stafford concluded, therefore, that constant email-checking is a kind of "normal" human behavior that includes *variable* reinforcement. Sometimes when we check our email, we get good news, and sometimes when we check it, we get bad news. Because we're not sure if a click on the email button will bring good news or bad, we tend to check our mailboxes often in the hopes of getting good news.

So what advice does Dr. Stafford give for users wanting to moderate this "normal" behavior pattern? The easiest fix, he said, is to weaken the *action* of clicking for the *receipt of a reward* (i.e., getting good news). Start with a five-minute delay between clicks and then increase the delay interval to thirty minutes or more. The longer the delay between clicks, the more likely you will get new email—and your much anticipated good news! Over time, you'll find checking your email will become less of a necessity.

Like email-checking, news-checking places in the "normal" end of behaviors rather than in the "concerning" end, because users tend to engage in this activity simply for information-gathering or entertainment. Apparently, news-checking addiction was first mentioned in 2012 by Professor Floyd Rudmin at the University of Tromso in Norway. What motivated him to investigate whether chronic news-checking is a problem was the large number of media pieces citing anecdotal evidence about self-identified news "junkies," who claimed that obsessive online news-checking interfered with their life routines. For example, one junkie confessed to checking a dozen different news sites every morning before thinking about getting going for the day. Though Professor Rudmin's research team developed a seven-item News Addiction Scale (NAS) to assess problematic news-checking, they quickly abandoned their research after finding that 70 percent of the population in Norway disclosed that they not only had a print newspaper subscription but also read news online daily. Professor Rudmin concluded that online news-reading appears to be a harmless habit helping users to become informed global citizens. It is not a behavior pattern requiring expert intervention.

Binge-watching addiction, the third type, is broadly defined as consecutively watching multiple episodes of a TV series in one sitting. Experts have suggested that this kind of activity would be viewed as problematic if it causes individuals to *regularly* have negative health consequences like lack of sleep, decreased exercise, impaired healthy eating, less effective day-to-day functioning at school or at work, and a reduced social life. So what is its prevalence in the general population? In 2019, Dr. Shreekantiah Umesh of the Central Institute of Psychiatry and Dr. Swarnali Bose of the Manipal Academy of Higher Education in India studied this issue and quickly concluded that while data indicate that binge-watching seems to be increasingly reported by users of all ages, its prevalence as an addiction rather than as a normal behavior is unlikely.

In fact, when all episodes of a TV season are released simultaneously by an online streaming service, entertainment-intensive marathon viewing is apparently widespread by users in all age categories, and particularly so in the teen and young adult age groups. Also, marathon viewers binge-watch and then post their reviews on SNSs for others in their virtual community to read. They also have conversations with virtual friends about these shows—saying that these increase their sense of belonging and well-being. In short, while marathon viewing seems to have more beneficial psychological consequences than harmful ones, there is a subset of higher-risk marathon viewers who tend to binge-watch alone and have no follow-up communications with others. These individuals often seek professional help because of their high degrees of experienced depression, loneliness, and poor self-regulation.

Let's focus now on two types of concerning behaviors: SNS addiction and IGD. Social media (or SNS) addiction has been defined by mental health experts as an inability to regulate one's own social media usage, leading to negative personal outcomes. In fact, an interesting 2018 US study by researchers Twenge, Joiner, and Rogers found that SNS engagement can be clinically problematic if usage exceeds one hour per day and quite possibly clinically addictive if usage exceeds two hours per day. So, given that online users in 2020 said that they spent an average of two hours and fifteen minutes per day on SNSs is concerning to experts because of the adverse impact this excessive behavior can have on users' longer-term well-being.

The reality is that there are positives and negatives affiliated with social media usage. On the plus side, particularly for teens and young adults, SNS connections help users maintain their relationships, seek new friendships with like-minded people, and escape from boredom. Unfortunately, because of these gratifications, users are at risk of addiction over the longer term. As publicly shared by *Facebook*'s Frances Haugen in her expert testimony in 2021, SNS platforms are, in fact, designed to keep users engaged often and for long periods of time to facilitate company profits.

In 2017, UK professors Daria Kuss and Mark Griffiths from Nottingham Trent University argued that SNS addiction is likely caused not just by a user's motivations for meeting certain social needs or by the platform's design features but by a combination of biological, psychological, and social factors known to exacerbate addictions. So what is it that SNS over-users likely become addicted to—the SNS technology itself and what it allows them to do, or something else? First, it seems that SNS users likely *do not* develop an addiction to the technology itself but to the rewards of being connected—such as the "Likes" received, the comments of appreciation obtained, and the growth in virtual friends. Second, it seems that SNS users have a "fear of missing out" (aka FOMO) about others' fun experiences if they are not routinely connected. Third, there appears to be a gender risk factor involved, such that females are more likely than males to fall victim to addiction, because they routinely spend more time on these platforms. Related to this third theme, there is growing evidence that SNS addiction in female teens often co-occurs with eating addiction and shopping addiction— two activities highly promoted by the ad sponsors on SNSs for this age group. Of major concern to mental health experts is that SNS-addicted females are more likely to report experiencing pronounced depressive symptoms, self-harm episodes, and suicide ideation or attempts.

If you are worried that you might be SNS-addicted, you can see a mental health professional to be assessed. You would be asked if you are experiencing these symptoms: (1) mood modifications—such that your SNS engagement changes your mood to a positive one from a negative one; (2) salience—such that you feel a combined behavioral, cognitive, and emotional preoccupation to engage in or tolerate more SNS activities; (3) withdrawal symptoms—such that you experience unpleasant physical and emotional symptoms when your SNS use is restricted or stopped; (4) conflict—such that you develop interpersonal and mental health problems because of your SNS over-usage; and (5) relapse—such that you revert to excessive SNS usage following any attempts to abstain from connecting.

Let's now turn to another very concerning online addiction reported by the American Psychiatric Association (APA) in 2013 and believed to be growing worse annually: IGD. Why, you may question, is online gaming considered to be so risky in terms of over-use or addiction? For starters, note the experts, online games have been designed to be seriously engaging for players, for they are built with detailed graphics, impressive visual stimuli, complicated plot sequences, and multiplayer capabilities. Because gamers are given a practically boundless license to explore themselves and others in a gaming virtual world before returning to the land-based real world, excessive gaming can become addictive because of the many gratifications it provides users.

Internet Gaming Disorder (IGD), sometimes called Internet Gaming Addiction (IGA), is defined by mental health experts to be the pathological playing of video games, resulting in harms to the player over the longer term. Individuals with IGD, in fact, share behavioral similarities with clients struggling with substance and gambling addiction. Also, teen males are more likely than teen females to be prone to this addiction. Why? Dr. Diane Wieland has posited that a prefrontal lobe predisposition in teen males' brains can lead to poor impulse control—which partly explains why IGD often co-occurs with problematic use of online pornography for this age group. Also, teen males tend to go online to fulfill an information glut, to play aggressive games with peers, or to engage in cybersex as they try to satisfy their needs for control, power, influence, and dominance. In contrast, teen females tend to go online to grow or maintain their friendships, to find romantic partners, or to seek emotional supports.

What's very concerning is that IGD, left untreated, can have dire consequences for users. One of the most dramatic and heavily publicized media stories regarding the perils of IGD harms occurred in 2005. Then, a 28-year-old South Korean man died after he played the game *StarCraft* at an internet cafe for fifty hours straight. He had not slept properly and had eaten very little in that time period. While no autopsy was ever done, he is believed to have died from heart failure stemming from exhaustion. In short, pathologic involvement in online gaming can result in users' experiencing neglect in several major life areas—including their school or work achievement, their self-care, and their land-based interpersonal relationships.

If you are concerned that you may be over doing your online gaming, at what point should you seek professional help? Game players at risk for addiction, affirm mental health experts, have many of these nine behaviors in common: (1) being preoccupied with your online gaming; (2) experiencing withdrawal symptoms if internet gaming is inaccessible or taken away from you; (3) experiencing tolerance issues, such that you feel a strong need to increase your time playing in order to be fulfilled; (4) being unsuccessful in your attempts to control online gaming; (5) having a loss of interest in your previously enjoyed land-based events and hobbies; (6) continuing your excessive use of online gaming, despite knowing you are already experiencing some psychological and/or social problems; (7) deceiving your family members or others about the amount of time you actually spend gaming; (8) having a tendency to relieve your negative moods by engaging in online gaming; and (9) having lost or feeling at risk of losing critical lifelines for maintaining your well-being, including your personal relationships and your achievements at school or at work. The bottom line is this: If you answered "yes" to at least five of these nine symptoms, you should consider seeking professional help.

4. How much screen time is considered healthy?

If you've wondered how much screen time is considered to be healthy, mental health experts say that the answer depends on the online platform you are talking about and your age. In fact, they argue, there is so much inconsistency in the definition of and the measurement of the various online addictions that even mental health experts themselves have difficulty ascertaining how much screen time is considered to be healthy or unhealthy on these various platforms. For this reason, in 2013, the APA reviewed how researchers and mental health professionals measured the various types of online addictions. Their conclusion was that the most consistency found in both definition and measurement was for online gaming addiction, or IGD.

However, psychiatrists caution that frequent or excessive online game playing *alone* does not serve as the basis for IGD diagnosis and therapeutic intervention, regardless of the amount of screen time reported. Rather, frequent and prolonged online game playing must cause *significant impairment* in *an individual's life*—such that the gamer plays compulsively to the exclusion of other formerly enjoyed life interests. Complicating the picture further is that IGD often co-occurs with problematic use of online pornography, particularly in adolescent males. A two-pronged addiction to online games and pornography by teen users, they warn, can lead to a very concerning deterioration in teens' land-based social skills and their relationship development, both particularly critical for maintaining well-being at this life stage.

As for healthy screen time regarding SNSs, recent reports—such as that produced by US experts Twenge, Joiner, and Rogers in 2018—indicate that SNS engagement can become clinically problematic if usage exceeds one hour per day and *possibly clinically addictive if usage exceeds two hours per day.* Again, a key factor to keep in mind here is that excessive SNS engagement becomes a legitimate mental health and well-being concern *only if it causes significant impairment in the user's life.*

Accepting that there seem to be no solid estimates at this time for what is considered to be an agreed-upon amount of healthy screen time, what pointers do mental health experts have for online users to help them safeguard their own well-being?

In 2020, psychiatrist Dr. Gary Small from the University of California cautioned that we have to be careful not to condemn online game playing or SNS engagement, per se, because both have benefits and risks to users. For example, online searching activities stimulate the neural activation of users' brain circuits controlling their decision-making and complex reasoning, and race car online gaming with distracting road signs has been found to hone gamers' multi-tasking skills. Also, action games have been found to improve users' visual attention, their reaction times, and their task-switching activities. On the downside, he notes, excessive screen time can heighten impulsivity in teen users, interfere with their emotional and social development, and result in addictive online behaviors. As a result, addicted users feel increasingly socially isolated, and they experience impaired sleep cycles and school achievement—particularly if their over-exposure is prolonged and other land-based life activities are downgraded or avoided altogether. The key, Dr. Small concludes, is to use the internet wisely and mindfully. If you as an online gamer or SNS engager have genuine concerns that your life is becoming unraveled because of your over-use, you are well advised to promptly seek a professional's assessment and possible treatment intervention.

5. What is FOMO, and how does it impact our use of technology?

Fear of missing out (or FOMO) on friends' daily life experiences has been found to be related to *both* SNS addiction and smartphone over-usage in teens, in particular. In the United States, alone, the proportion of teens aged 13–17 who now own smartphones is a significant 89 percent. In fact, the rate of phone ownership in this age group has doubled here in just six years! So it is not surprising that smartphone ownership and SNS engagement go hand-in-hand. In fact, about 70 percent of teens admit to connecting to SNSs multiple times a day, typically through their smartphones. Furthermore, smartphone over-usage has been associated with an increase in a phenomenon called "nomophobia," the clinical name given by mental health experts to someone having an intense fear of being without or away from one's phone.

The term "nomophobia"—short form for "no mobile phone phobia"—was coined in 2008 by the UK's post office in a study completed there. Users having this fear are known to worry when they're unable to use their phones, are known to check them often, may never turn their phones off—even at bedtime or throughout the night, and may carry an extra phone charger in their purses or backpacks. In this study, 58 percent of male respondents and 48 percent of female respondents reportedly suffered from considerable distress when their phones were switched off, and a significant 55 percent of the respondents said that the main reason for their phobia was not being able to maintain contact with their loved ones.

While smartphone users today experience various degrees of nomophobia, mental health experts believe that the driving factors for this condition include FOMO, boredom, loneliness, and personal insecurities. So how would you know if you are a nomophobic? In 2016, Dr. Narendra Kumar Pathak, an academic counselor at Indira Gandhi National University in India, said that nomophobic symptoms include these experiences: (1) a lack of concentration, (2) a feeling of irritation if you are separated from your phone or when the phone's battery is running low, (3) a strong urge by you to look at your phone first thing in the morning and the last thing at night—often interfering with a restful sleep pattern, (4) a tendency for you to ignore (or phub) other people present while being immersed in your phone, and (5) a noticeable reduction in your productivity at school or work because of an overwhelming need to be connected to your phone, often accompanied by an overwhelming sense of FOMO. So, if you have determined that these experiences describe you well, chances, he says, you are a nomophobic.

In 2017, UK professor Dr. Mark Griffiths affirmed that nomophobia is rooted in an intense fear of not being able to engage in social connections. So owning a smartphone gives teens the ability to join an SNS like *Facebook* or *Twitter* 24/7 to feel forever connected to their virtual and land-based friends. It is along this line of thinking, he posits, that there exists a theoretical association between nomophobia and SNS addiction. So what are the reported downsides to being a nomophobic? Dr. Griffiths and his colleague Daria Kuss affirm that constant tethering to one's smartphone can produce a series of unexpected negative personal consequences for users, including impaired social interactions on land and a vast array of body and mental health problems. This list of harms includes digital eye strain, "tech neck," anxiety, depression, and elevated levels of stress—driven by a growing sense that one is lacking in real "quality" relationships, resulting in increased social isolation. Over the longer term, social isolation has been linked to poor health and premature mortality. Finally, nomophobia can lead to users' relying on and using their smartphones in impulsive ways—contributing to SNS over-usage or addiction.

How prevalent is nomophobia in teens and young adults? In 2021, Dr. Venetia Notara from the University of West Attica in Greece tried to answer this question by completing a systematic review of studies addressing nomophobia in the 18–25-year age group. She concluded that the prevalence of this phenomenon ranged widely from a low of 15.2 percent to a high of 99.7 percent for this age group, depending on geographic location and affordable smartphone accessibility.

6. Can overusing technology cause or worsen anxiety, depression, and other mental health conditions?

Nowadays, while a certain amount of online screen time is necessary to complete tasks for school or work and to connect with friends or play online games, users routinely overusing technology can create adverse mental health conditions for themselves. While experts caution us to mindfully limit our screen time on all digital devices to two hours daily, they acknowledge that some users are more likely than others to develop an online addiction—based on known factors like age, gender, cultural norms, personality, and genetics. So how can you determine if you are dangerously overusing technology?

Let's take a closer look at two key warning signs that you should view as over-use "red flags." First, are you routinely experiencing signs of *depression*—with your days and/or nights marked by negativity, apathy, or withdrawal from your previously enjoyed land-based activities? Second, are you routinely experiencing signs of *anxiety*—with your days and/or nights marked by edginess, sleeplessness, or moodiness?

How do experts define depression and anxiety? For starters, it is important to note that it is not life events, per se, that create a sense of anxiety or depression in individuals but *an individual's appraisal* of life events in the land-based or virtual world. For depression, an individual's appraisal often relates to a perceived loss regarding a coveted relationship, one's status among coworkers or friends, or one's competence at school or work. As a label, "depression" is used by experts in a number of ways—to describe a mood, a syndrome, or an illness (known as a clinical disorder).

As a mood, depression is part of a normal range of life experiences. As a syndrome, it consists of a depressed mood—along with outward signs of distress, such as noticeable weight loss, weight gain, or an inability to concentrate for extended periods. As a clinical disorder, depression involves *both* a syndrome of depression and an implication it is not transitory in nature—and that it causes significant impairment in the individual's well-being. This point needs to be underscored: *Clinical disorders of depression are curable only with the help of a mental health professional.*

Now let's focus on anxiety. In anxiety, an individual's thoughts tend to center on some perceived physical or psychological danger in the land-based or the virtual world. Anxiety is also part of a normal range of life experiences. As a mood, it can be fleeting or chronic. Individuals with chronic states of anxiety tend to routinely overestimate the "real dangers" in their life, and for this reason, *chronic anxiety sufferers often seek professional help to reduce their unrelenting discomfort.*

Mental health professionals assisting clients experiencing chronic anxiety further differentiate between two broad types of clinical anxiety, each requiring unique treatment plans. The first is "recurrent panic attacks," considered to be a rather ineffective stress coping mechanism relied upon by individuals in high-distress situations. The second is "generalized anxiety disorder," a personality disorder involving unrealistic or excessive worry caused by life circumstances over an extended period of time.

In recurrent panic attacks, individuals tend to experience a sudden, intense feeling of apprehension or impending doom, leading them to think that they are having a heart attack, are losing control, or might be experiencing some form of short-term insanity. Because by their very nature panic attacks are generally unpredictable in terms of their onset, not knowing when the next one will occur adds to the individual's distress. The good news is that a form of psychotherapy known as cognitive behavioral therapy (CBT), is an effective intervention used by professionals that results in long-term symptom relief and more effective stress-coping in their clients.

Finally, in generalized anxiety disorder, distressed individuals routinely experience a wide range of uncomfortable mental and physical symptoms— such as muscle tension, breathlessness, fatigue, sweating, nausea, diarrhea, sleep disturbances, difficulty concentrating, irritability, and so on. Although thoughts associated with this form of excessive worry vary, they generally involve a rather broad appraisal by the individual of not being able to cope with a series of current life circumstances. The good news is that there are forms of psychotherapy that are very effective at not only reducing these uncomfortable symptoms for individuals but helping them to construct more effective stress-coping mechanisms over the longer term.

7. What is appearance-related social media consciousness, and how can it impact your mental health?

Social Networking Site (SNS) frequent users report having a FOMO on others' fun life experiences if they are not routinely connected. For this reason, mental health experts say that there appears to be a gender risk factor for SNS addiction, because teen females routinely spend more time on these platforms and on their smartphones, compared to their male peers. Also, teen females' social life and status maintenance often revolve around intimacy and inclusion—or fear of exclusion—more so than for males. This fear of exclusion also contributes to their propensity to fall prey to "appearance-related consciousness" or "social media consciousness"—defined as the extent to which females' thoughts and behaviors reflect a strong need to look attractive to their social media audience.

Generally speaking, appearance-related consciousness applies to users looking to social media for feedback and/or validation of themselves as an "interesting human being." Consequently, these users tend to focus on how many "Likes" or comments a post of theirs (often their own photo) receives on their favored SNS. While on the surface, focusing on this feedback aspect of SNS engagement appears to be innocent and non-threatening, mental health experts have cautioned that this kind of external validation of self-worth can harm a young person's self-esteem, especially those having low social-emotional well-being.

These mental health harms typically involve a psychological process known as "an upward social comparison." Simply put, SNS users engaged in routine feedback-seeking compare themselves to someone that they perceive to be superior in some way—often a celebrity, an "influencer," or a socially popular peer. In the end, the SNS heavy user concludes that she (or he) falls miserably short on some desired trait—whether it is weight or beauty—causing her (or him) to become increasingly dissatisfied with themselves.

Mental health professionals affirm that both female and male clients seeking treatment often express feeling intense dissatisfaction with their body image and appearance—leaving them feeling depressed, anxious, less confident, and very unhappy. Some engage in suicide ideation or practice self-harm. Others develop disordered eating habits, with males tending to "bulk up" and with females tending to "lose weight."

How much SNS-browsing is considered by mental health experts to possibly lead to social media consciousness? While the verdict is still out on this issue, in one recent study, female participants reported experiencing more negative moods *after just ten minutes* of browsing *Facebook* accounts that were curated or digitally altered, compared with female participants browsing appearance-neutral websites. In short, say mental health experts, the very nature of social media interactions—which are at arm's length and often anonymous—makes negative commenting about other users' appearance easy and harsher than comments typically made in land-based interactions. In fact, it is this anonymity of online commenting that has likely contributed to SNS users' exaggerated concerns about appearance and status among peers.

So, how can you protect yourself from such SNS-induced harms? Dr. Gary Goldfield, a Canadian mental health expert, affirms "that less is better." He posits that female and male teens feel better about their appearance and body weight after they cut their use of social media in half for three weeks—to an average of 78 minutes a day from around 189 minutes a day.

Finally, mental health experts warn that SNS business practices aimed at generating profits at users' expense add to the "SNS harms mix." Specifically, ads placed on targeted SNSs tend to focus on the most vulnerable, low self-esteem users. What's equally as damaging, these advertisers often suggest that their many featured products and services provide "quick fixes" for users' shortcomings—from make-up, to skin care, to brands of clothing—and are, therefore, the perfect recipe for increased peer inclusion and happiness. Sadly, the reality is that this business practice further undermines teens' self-confidence and feelings of self-worth when the products or services purchased fail to meet their hyped-up expectations.

To better safeguard SNS users, democratic governments globally have either passed or are in the process of passing legislation to curb these harm-inducing phenomena. For example, in 2021, Norway passed a law requiring SNS "influencers" to label heavily edited or retouched photos on social media—or to risk paying a sizable fine and/or serving jail time. The UK is currently working on a Digitally Altered Body Images Bill that would require paid "influencers" to label posts where an image of a human body or body part has been digitally altered.

8. What kinds of psychological or psychiatric conditions are typically found in people who over-use technology?

Mental health experts warn that over-using technology can lead to increased levels of depression and anxiety in online users. In fact, these two negative moods are typically reported by users *not mindful* of their excessive usage of their digital devices over extended periods of time. Experts also warn that with excessive use of screen time and online gaming, in particular, any pre-existing condition in gamers related to attention-deficit/hyperactivity disorder (ADHD)—characterized by an excess of hyperactive, inattentive, and impulsive behaviors in users—can be exacerbated. But why does this happen?

Disinhibition, defined by mental health practitioners as a failure by an individual to suppress inappropriate responding to, say, "a go" or "no-go" life task seems to be central in determining if an avid online user or gamer has ADHD. In fact, of the three disorders known to be related to technology over-use—depression, anxiety, and ADHD—the latter is a more common psychiatric disorder diagnosed in teens also having internet addiction.

Again, you may ask, "Why?" Professionals believe that several rather complex bio-psycho-social mechanisms might explain the coexistence of ADHD and IGD, particularly in males. Since online gaming is generally characterized by rapid responses and (hopefully) immediate rewards for users, the online environment may provide immediate stimulation and rewards for individuals with ADHD, known to become easily bored and have an aversion to delayed rewards.

Three key reasons offered by mental health experts for the coexistence between ADHD and IGD in teens and adolescents include these: (1) since most individuals with ADHD tend to be attracted to enhanced simulations with quick reward paths, online games with their "get to the next game level" incentives present a very attractive reward path for teen players with ADHD; (2) because individuals with ADHD commonly have abnormal brain activities associated with impaired inhibition and difficulty in controlling or limiting their internet use, they are particularly susceptible to online game addiction, relative to their peers not experiencing ADHD symptoms; (3) because ADHD symptoms can negatively impact interpersonal relationships, these individuals may choose to form social relationships in the virtual world rather than in the land-based world.

How prevalent is the occurrence of ADHD with anxiety and depression in teens? Recent studies have reported that over a third of teens and adolescents with ADHD suffer from anxiety, with generalized anxiety disorder being the most prevalent. Also, anywhere from 5 percent to 40 percent of adolescents with ADHD also suffer from major depression. Finally, the risk of internet addiction and IGD, combined, is associated with an increased prevalence of substance or drug dependence in online users.

9. How does technology over-use negatively impact relationships in real life?

Though on face it may seem counterintuitive to you, a number of recent studies have reported that excessive social media use or online gaming use is linked with *social isolation*—with over-users more likely to feel as though they do not have enough good quality relationships, compared to light or moderate users. If you are concerned that this perception applies to you, mental health experts warn that if social isolation is left undiagnosed and untreated, the long-term prognosis is not positive. Extended feelings of social isolation in online users have been associated with a number of negative consequences over the longer term—such as poor health outcomes, increased pornography use, increased substance abuse (including drugs and alcohol), and increased morbidity and mortality.

So how much social isolation is too much? An interesting 2017 study conducted by Brian Primack and colleagues at the University of Pittsburgh found that for the segment of the approximately 1,800 study participants aged 19–32 years who admitted to engaging in social media for *two or more hours daily*, they had double the odds of experiencing social isolation compared with peers who limited their social media use to less than thirty minutes daily.

Some possible explanations offered by this US research team included not only considerable reductions in rewarding land-based social experiences for these social media over-users but an increase in their tendency to make upward social comparisons based on social media feeds and "Likes" received. For the most part, warn mental health professionals, such error-filled types of feedback produce unrealistic expectations about how online users should be in real life. What's more, receiving a daily dose of negative feedback tends to provoke insecurities around online users' self-adequacy—triggering repeat cycles of social isolation over time. Put simply, these online users would likely rather run the risk of becoming socially isolated than run the risk of being socially rejected by peers because they are "so imperfect."

To reduce the harms of increasing social isolation, mental health experts say that users would be well advised to be assessed by a mental health professional if they think they are at risk. There is a clinical intervention technique known as cognitive behavioral therapy (CBT) that has proven to be very effective in helping social media over-users break the cycle of social isolation (described more fully in question 49).

10. What is phubbing?

How does it make you feel when you are actively engaged in a conversation with someone and all of a sudden that person pulls out the smartphone and starts texting, ignoring you? Angry? Deflated? Rejected? You have just experienced what is called "phubbing." A decade ago, on the stopphubbing website (still active today), the term "phubbing"—actually a portmanteau of the words *phone* and *snubbing*—described the act of paying attention to your smartphone instead of talking to the person directly in your company.

The history of phubbing as a phenomenon is quite interesting. Saurav Pathak, a management professor at Kansas State University, says that the term was originally coined in a campaign by the *Macquarie Dictionary* to represent a growing problem of smartphone over-use and misuse in social settings. By definition, "a phubber" is the person phubbing his or her companion, while "a phubbee" is the person receiving the phubbing behavior.

So how prevalent is phubbing in present-day social situations? In an interesting 2015 study completed by Lee Ranie and Kathryn Zickuhr from the Pew Research Center in Washington, DC, a whopping 90 percent of the study respondents said that not only did they engage in phubbing during recent social activities, but that they were phubbed an equal number of times by others. Apparently this lack of social etiquette appears to be commonplace in today's connected society. In terms of romantic interactions and phubbing frequency, another study completed in 2016 by James Roberts and Meredith David from the Baylor University Business School found that nearly half of adult respondents said they were regularly phubbed by their romantic partners.

What are the likely predictors of phubbing? In 2016, British researchers Varoth Chotpitayasunondh and Karen Douglass from the University of Kent School of Psychology tried to shed some light on this question. Their research found that the most important determinant of phubbing appears to be smartphone over-use or addiction. The more distant predictors of phubbing seem to be internet addiction, FOMO on friends' social activities, and a lack of social etiquette or poor impulse control by phubbers. These researchers added that the phubbing behavior itself determines the extent to which people are phubbed. In other words, being a phubber results in a vicious, self-reinforcing cycle of phubbing that makes this rather objectionable social interaction activity seem more normative.

Finally, a number of negative social consequences affiliated with phubbing have been documented. Perceived harms by phubbees include experiencing: (1) negative, resentful reactions, such that social interactions with others are perceived to be of lower quality; (2) reduced levels of trust in partners; (3) increased social-emotional distance from partners—particularly when a smartphone is present; and (4) jealousy and deflated mood following social interactions with one's partner. These negative consequences, say mental health experts, represent a form of social exclusion—or ostracism—that threatens our basic human needs and leads to deflated affect in victims. Ostracism is defined as "feeling excluded from the social interactions of those around us, leaving us with emotional feelings of aggression, anxiety, depression, and loneliness." Being ostracized also threatens our longer-term needs to belong, for self-esteem, for meaningful existence, and for self-control.

Phubbers—whether or not they are consciously aware of the personal harms they cause others—are "guilty" of breaking social etiquette protocols by rejecting phubbees' needs: (1) to belong by demonstrating explicitly or symbolically that they are not wanted or valued in the partnership; (2) or self-esteem and self-control by punishing them—leading to a sense of their feeling unworthy to receive others' attention; and (3) for meaningful existence by producing in them a sense of "social death" or invisibility. Consequently, to avoid such negative feelings and a woeful lack of basic human need fulfillment, phubees may self-impose their own social isolation over the longer term.

In short, caution mental health experts, what appears on the surface to be a rather harmless, commonplace activity, phubbing has some rather substantial psychological harms associated with these acts that users should be mindful of when interacting with others in our virtual/land-based hybrid social environments.

11. How does technology over-use negatively impact academic performance?

Smartphones, with their pervasive acceptance and powerful functionality, have without a doubt become an integral part of our daily activities. While in 2018, the Pew Research Center found that 95 percent of university students used their smartphones to function at school and for leisure, during the Covid-19 lockdowns, smartphone usage was projected to be nearly 100 percent for students across grade levels. So how does technology over-usage negatively impact students' academic performance—if at all?

According to mental health experts, there is a downside to intense usage of technology over time, with documented negative consequences impacting users' well-being. Reported negative aspects include users' feeling socially isolated, highly anxious, and unable to maintain positive sleep or eating routines. For students, an over-reliance on technology daily has reportedly not only impaired their learning activities and academic performance but caused myriad physical and mental symptoms, such as blurred vision, wrist pain, insomnia, next-day fatigue, and depression.

Are there any known steps that students can take to moderate the negative impact of technology over-usage on their learning and well-being during high-stress periods? To answer this question, in 2021 a research team led by Professor Fu of the School of Information Management at Wuhan University in China posited that the positive aspects of health information literacy—which emphasizes the positive role of health information in optimizing individuals' *mindful* self-care—should be studied to gain insights into how it could help students during high-stress periods. Simply put, health information literacy is the degree to which users can obtain and process health information for making sound lifestyle decisions to alleviate known harms. This team's research focused on the particular role health literacy could play in moderating the negative outcomes of smartphone over-use by nearly 7,000 Chinese university students surveyed during the Covid-19 pandemic.

What were their key study findings and well-being takeaways, as reported by these students? First, smartphone over-use during this time was strongly associated with students' increased deterioration in sleep quality (caused by later bedtimes and blue light sleep disturbances), insomnia, nomophobia (i.e., fear of being separated from their phones), and rapid deterioration in their eyesight (i.e., cellphone vision syndrome). Second, smartphone over-use had a significant adverse impact on students' academic performance and daytime learning, exacerbated by the just-cited symptoms. For example, nomophobia (manifested as chronically texting others during the academic day) became a needless distraction in the virtual classroom, hindering students' lesson focus. Also, poor eyesight prevented many students from gaining knowledge effectively, and ongoing insomnia decreased their seven-hour refueling sleep time needed for overnight recovery. Third, while health information literacy played a moderating positive role by helping many students to mindfully limit their smartphone usage before and during bedtime to reduce insomnia and poor eyesight, it *did not* moderate the pandemic-enhanced relationship between smartphone over-use and nomophobia. Fourth, while health literacy was somewhat effective for the bulk of students to help them maintain their well-being and academic performance during these high-stress periods, it was deemed to be quite ineffective for students previously clinically assessed as having some form of internet addiction.

A key "takeaway" from this study, note the researchers, is this: When students are concerned about their declining well-being and academic performance during high-stress periods—especially when known "mindful" health literacy steps have been implemented but failed to fully remedy their issues, they should seek additional guidance and more holistic interventions from a mental health professional.

12. How does technology over-use negatively impact employment and job performance?

If you've wondered how workplace technology usage impacts employees' job performance and their work-life balance, a series of business studies have recently provided considerable clarity on this complex front. On the plus side of the productivity equation, technology usage has provided new opportunities for employees to stay connected via email or Zoom meetings at short notice and at all times of the day or night. In fact, during the Covid-19 lockdowns, online platforms like *Google Meet* and *Zoom* allowed employees to work from home and not miss a critical work deadline. More recently, generative Artificial Intelligence (AI) deployment shows solid potential for taking over routine aspects of many jobs—saving organizations time and resources—and allowing employees to apply their special skills, critical thinking, and high-level knowledge to important aspects of the job where AI is not necessarily a value-add.

Recent research on the over-use of technology by employees has also provided some clarity on the negative side of the productivity equation. For example, in 2017, Stoney Brooks from Middle Tennessee State University found that when employees routinely viewed *Facebook* or *YouTube* as a workplace distraction, their levels of social media "techno-stress" grew from an entertainment nicety at work to a real susceptibility to develop internet addiction. Simply put, techno-stress is workplace stress caused by an excessive use of Information and Communication Technologies (ICTs). Also, in 2019, workplace consultants Tawaziwa Wushe and Jacob Shenje found that government employees' time routinely spent on social media applications like *Twitter*, *WhatsApp*, and *Facebook* had a significant negative relationship on their productivity and job performance.

So how do the positives of technology use at work turn into a productivity nightmare for employees? In 2021, Montressa Washington from Shenandoah University in Virginia tried to answer this question. By taking what is called a socio-technical approach (defined as the interaction between the technical and social subsystems at work) to her study design, this professor evaluated the impact on employees of information overload at work, their ability to self-regulate technology usage on and off the job, how work overload impacted their relationships with family members, and how technology addiction affected their work productivity. She reasoned that though smartphones, computers, and meeting apps like *Zoom* can augment employees' work productivity by allowing them to not only be connected with others in the workplace during working hours but immediately responsive to workplace task deadlines or emergencies after working hours, these provisions could also promote a series of negative outcomes over the longer term, if sustained, including technology addiction, work overload/ burnout, and work-life imbalances.

To test her hypotheses, an online survey was distributed to 300 full-time working professionals in the United States who routinely used digital technologies to accomplish their workplace goals. In total, there were 145 male and 155 female respondents, mostly employed in firms classified as private and for profit (68 percent). The respondents represented both non-management

(54 percent) and management positions (46 percent), with the majority of them (72 percent) ranging in age from twenty-six to fifty-four years.

Key study findings provided important insights into how technology overuse can impact employees' workplace performance, including these three: (1) employees with technology addictions early on had significantly lower workplace productivity in the short- and long-term; (2) employees' work overloads, if sustained but not a problem initially, interfered significantly with their family life and work-life balance over the longer term and were positively related to their being at risk for developing a technology addiction; and (3) employees' inability to self-regulate their technology usage in the short- and long-term was negatively related to their workplace productivity and was positively related to their eventually developing a technology addiction.

Given these rather alarming findings, Professor Washington affirmed that workplace wellness programs should encourage employees experiencing technology addiction or an inability to self-regulate technology usage to seek mental health assistance provided by their organizations. In fact, accepting that technology is ubiquitous in today's workplaces, employers should promote work-life balance by rewarding employees achieving a "mindful" balance between their workplace productivity and family life fulfillment. For companies not advocating this stance, legislation promoting "the right to disconnect" after hours is bound to fill this void.

13. Is technology use always bad for mental and social health?

There is little question that the digital revolution continues to change our world and our lives. We saw how in the repeat Covid-19 pandemic lockdowns, technology use enabled students to facilitate their learning without leaving home and employees to complete their work requirements remotely. But there were also some reported downsides to extensive technology use and relationship health during the Covid-19 pandemic. Let's look more closely at this outcome.

When working adults suddenly found themselves facing extended lockdowns and daily online tethering, they had to quickly adapt to new realities on the home front, including having to spend much more time than usual at home with their spouse, their children, and their pets. For some people, this change in work-life routine may have provided them with a great opportunity to strengthen their family bonds. But for others, it was perceived to be a very painful mental and relationship experience—causing some spouses to consider or to undergo divorce proceedings.

The present-day reality of "hybrid" workplaces (involving both in-home and at-work phases) raises the intriguing question: Is technology over-usage bad for mental and relationship health in most adults? Also, are certain age groups particularly vulnerable to experiencing such harms?

In an attempt to address these important questions, in 2020, a research team led by Margret Hoehe at the Max Planck Institute for Molecular Genetics in Berlin, Germany, reviewed ten related study findings and concluded that there is ample evidence indicating that digital technology may influence our brains, our mental health, and our relationships in both negative and positive ways at various life stages. Let's take a closer look at how and why.

Two key themes emerged from this multi-study review. First, brain imaging techniques show that critical brain changes in early childhood and during adolescence occur, impacting our skill and relationship development capabilities. Some of these brain changes are negatively related to the effects of digital media use on mental health and relationships, while others are positively related. Second, the Covid-19 pandemic, in particular, has recharged the debate among mental health experts about whether humans at all life stages who are tethered to their computers and smartphones for whatever reason (such as school or work) are just not "natural" at any life stage primarily because tethering hampers our land-based relationship building.

Let's drill down into the evidence along these two key themes, beginning with the negative and positive factors associated with excessive screen time exposure in preschoolers and adolescents and their relationship development. For parents who think that allowing their preschoolers to have full access to computers or other digital devices because it will aid in their cognitive and relationship development may find it surprising to learn that magnetic resonance imaging (MRI) findings have consistently shown that screen over-exposure in preschoolers impairs the brain's white matter development supporting language, literacy, and relationship-building skills [a definite negative factor].

Adolescence is also a time of significant brain development in areas involving emotional and social behavior. In particular, there is considerable evidence that the density of gray matter in the amygdala—a structure associated with emotional processing—is important during this life stage. There is an interplay between gray matter density and social experiences gained in both virtual and land-based environments. In other words, for adolescents to effectively gain critical relationship-building skills that will last them throughout their lifetimes, online social experiences *should not replace* critical off-line social experiences but rather *complement* them [a positive factor].

Comprehensive studies assessing the negative effects of excessive screen time on adolescents' brains have also involved the neurological and biological mechanisms related to online gaming addiction, per se. These studies have consistently revealed through brain imaging results that clinically diagnosed teen game addicts have many of the negative brain alterations seen in other substance (i.e., drug and alcohol) addicts. Specifically, there are concerning patterns of brain activation in regions associated with impairment in teens' cognitive, motor, and sensory functions—all of which are needed for positive relationship building during this important life stage [a negative factor].

Now let's look at the second key theme around excessive technology use and its effects on humans' mental and relationship development at all life stages. Both before and after the Covid-19 tethering experience, there has been a strongly expressed view among many mental health experts that there is something about the whole phenomenon of being digitally tethered for extended periods of time that is just not "natural" for humans. These experts posit that humans did not evolve to be staring at digital screens for much of their waking or sleeping hours. Rather, they evolved to interact with others face-to-face on a daily basis and to use their senses of smell, touch, taste, sight, and sound to secure their work-life balance as well as their relationships. They further maintain that for humans to optimize our mental and relationship health over the longer term, we need to take a routine break from technology both in normative and in stressful times.

There is another smaller faction of mental health experts, however, who argue that humans have evolved to appreciate the natural allure of digital media. They maintain that the intensive technology use seen during adolescence, in particular, is part of humans' grand evolutionary design to help them better cope with life and relationship challenges at any life stage. In short, the debate currently underway among mental health experts over the pluses and minuses of technology use at various life stages and its impact on individuals' development and relationship building will remain active for the foreseeable future.

The Negative Impact of Technology Over-Use on Physical Health and Safety

14. What is digital eye strain?

The recent Covid-19 pandemic led to an increase in complaints by digital device users about eye strain and headaches. What exactly is digital eye strain, and how can it be effectively dealt with? Digital eye strain (DES) or computer vision syndrome (CVS) was defined in 2020 by the American Optometric Association (AOA) to include a range of visual and ocular symptoms caused by prolonged use of computers, tablets, e-readers, and smartphones. According to these eye experts, looking at a digital screen for long periods of time *without taking a break* makes the eyes work harder, resulting in their becoming susceptible to developing the vision-related symptoms of DES. In fact, digital device users with uncorrected vision problems before the pandemic had an increased susceptibility to develop more severe DES symptoms during it.

So what is it that makes digital device viewing more difficult for the eyes than when reading from a printed page? Compared to the printed page, the letters on a digital device are not as precise or as sharply defined, the level of contrast of letters relative to the screen background is reduced, and the presence of glare and screen reflections make viewing more challenging for the eyes. Also, digital device users must view distances and angles for screen work differently than when reading from a printed page. As a result, eye-focusing attempts and eye movements place increased stress demands on the eyes. In fact, users who previously suffered from minor vision problems before the pandemic lockdowns complained about more pronounced visual discomfort and decreased eye performance when tethered to their screens for hours on end, day after day.

Individuals with an eyeglass or contact lens prescription already in place prior to tethering found that their existing lens correction was just not suitable for the viewing distances required by screens, so they were prone to tilt their heads at odd angles for lengthy periods. Also, they tended to bend toward their screens for extended periods to see the letters and images more clearly—resulting in agonizing muscle spasms or pain in their necks, shoulders, or backs.

Generally speaking, individuals spending *two or more continuous hours* at a computer or digital screen daily are not only at risk for developing DES but also experiencing symptoms such as eyestrain, headaches, blurred vision, dry eyes, and neck and shoulder pain. These symptoms may be caused by or exacerbated by a number of environmental factors as well, including poor lighting, glare on a screen, improper viewing distances, poor seating posture, and uncorrected vision problems. The good news is that many of these symptoms are temporary and will decrease with smart digital device use. Also, device users' eye doctors may suggest some changes for implementation regarding how the screen is viewed, whether special digital device eyeglasses should be prescribed, or if existing prescriptions should be adjusted.

The AOA gives these useful pointers to help digital device users reduce the onset or worsening of DES symptoms: (1) minimize eye discomforts from blue light and glare by employing a glare reduction filter, repositioning the screen, or using drapes or blinds in the work area; (2) adjust the study or work area for comfort by placing the computer screen 20 to 30 inches away from you and making sure that the top of the screen is slightly below your horizontal eye level; (3) use an adjustable copyholder to place your reading material at the same distance from your eyes as the computer screen and as close as possible to the screen; and (4) take task breaks throughout the day by making phone calls or walking about for some time to help your eyes rest and to not have to focus on something up-close.

15. What is "tech neck"?

Have you experienced a sore neck after hunching over your computer screen or smartphone for hours on end to complete school assignments, remote work, or connect with friends? If so, you are suffering from what is known as "tech neck," and given current stats on smartphone usage/over-usage, you are likely not alone. In 2021, there were over 290 million smartphone users in the United States—suggesting that 85 percent of Americans now regularly talk, read, text, scroll, or tap their smartphones daily, and Statista projects that the average American will spend on average four hours and thirty-five continuous minutes daily on their smartphones in 2023—definitely over the two-hour safety threshold recommended by the AOA for eye health maintenance.

What exactly is "tech neck," and how can it be relieved or prevented? The American Massage Therapy Association (AMTA) refers to this neck condition as being caused by individuals' hunching over a computer or a smartphone screen while holding their shoulder girdle in a less than an ideal position, or by holding their heads unnaturally far forward to stare at their computer or phone monitors. Technically, these unnatural postures cause repetitive strain and injury, resulting in symptoms such as neck pain, upper back pain, chronic headaches, and increased curvature of the spine. In terms of symptom intensity, tech neck sufferers have described their sore body parts as ranging from a chronic nagging discomfort to an agonizing sharp, stabbing, localized pain.

The AMTA says that while tech neck is caused by several overstretched, fatigued muscles in both the neck and upper back, one muscle particularly affected is the sternocleidomastoid (SCM). The SCM functions by binding our skull to our sternum and clavicle, with its anchoring point in front of our body and the attachment point in the back of our head. The SCM typically pulls our head forward and tilts our head into extension. It is most often linked to tech neck because of the "unnatural" prolonged, frequent, forward head, and hunched shoulder postures we adopt to use our digital devices.

Besides the neck and back muscles, nerves can also be adversely impacted by ongoing shoulder hunching—with the occipital neuralgia being particularly affected. These nerves typically exit the spine at the base of the neck and thread their way up the neck's back and through several muscles before reaching the skull. Tense neck muscles put extra pressure on the occipital nerves, exacerbating the tech neck syndrome and intensifying painful symptoms in users.

Over the longer term, as users' muscles tighten, shorten, lengthen, and take on new positions, they unfortunately "forget" their purpose as intended by nature. That's when muscle atrophy results, requiring tech neck sufferers to register for massage therapy to restore the muscles to their intended purpose and health. The good news is that this condition responds well to muscle release techniques known as Myofascial Release (MFR). With MFR, the massage therapist puts light, sustained pressure on targeted fascia connective tissue to reduce the pain and to restore muscle strength and motion. This therapy combines active isolated stretching with light pressure over the adversely impacted muscle groups. Also, therapists often use trigger point therapy to help heal the anterior (front) muscles; they are "softened" by the therapist's putting pressure on the knots in the muscle fiber contributing to the neck pain.

Can tech neck be prevented? Studies have shown that timely interventions by massage therapists for the tech neck pain—along with users' sound knowledge about the importance of taking frequent breaks from "unnatural" hunched postures while on our digital devices are key to not only treating the condition once it appears but also preventing it from beginning in the first place.

16. How does over-using technology negatively affect sleep?

How often do you get the recommended seven hours of sleep per night for optimal functioning the next day? If you replied, "not often enough," you are in good company. Sleep experts allege that a high proportion of adolescents and adults are chronically sleep-deprived because of their over-usage of technology. Eventually, these sleep-deprived sufferers arrive at their medical clinics for treatment because of their poor cognitive control, reduced academic performance, and reduced socio-emotional functioning.

How bad is the problem of sleep deprivation? In 2017, prior to the Covid-19 pandemic, a US research team led by psychology professor Jean Twenge at San Diego State University said that even then over 40 percent of adolescents reportedly slept less than the recommended seven hours a night, in large part, because their smartphone and technology usage far exceeded the recommended two hours of screen time daily recommended by mental health professionals.

Researchers have also found that adolescents' and adults' regular use of blue-light-emitting smartphones before bedtime disrupts their sleep quality and duration in many ways. It takes longer for users to fall asleep, decreases their healthy evening sleepiness factor, and reduces their melatonin secretion or "calming sleep hormone" (produced naturally by the pineal gland). Other reported sleep deficiencies because of tech over-use before bedtime include a circadian clock delay, reduced amounts and quality of "self-healing" rapid eye movement (REM) sleep, and markedly reduced alertness levels the next morning. Yet another bad tech habit users are guilty of is their temptation to carry their smartphones into the bedroom so they can check for "important" texts or emails throughout the night rather than take part in uninterrupted self-healing sleep.

It is one thing to have disrupted sleep problems every now and then, caution the experts, but if sleeping fewer than seven hours a night becomes a habit over the longer term, there are serious mental health issues that can emerge—including depressed mood, reduced self-esteem, poor stress coping, and increased risk for internet addiction. The "bottom line," say these experts, is that digital device users not only need to be *mindful* of the importance of routinely getting enough restful sleep to stay healthy and mood-balanced but should forego screen viewing *at least an hour or more* before bedtime. Also, screen viewing should not routinely occur during bedtime. Stated simply, your smartphone is *not your bedroom buddy* and should not accompany you to bed! Leave it in another room overnight, and don't get up to read any text messages or emails until the next morning. If you need an alarm to wake you in a timely fashion, consider investing in an old-fashioned alarm clock instead of relying on your blue light-emitting smartphone.

17. What other ways can technology over-use negatively impact your physical health?

Besides tech neck, sleep disruptions, mood dysfunction, and various types of technology addictions, technology over-use can negatively impact users' health, including lowering their levels of much-needed physical activity and raising their propensity for accidents.

What can users do to reduce these negatives regarding physical health? Let's start with the amount of physical activity experts say we need routinely to maintain our well-being and reduce our accident propensity. According to the World Health Organization (WHO) guidelines, children, adolescents, and adults should engage in at least 75 minutes of vigorous physical activity per week, at least 150 minutes of moderate physical activity, or any equivalent combination of the two. So, if you're falling far short of this target because of technology over-use, this sedentary behavior should serve as a "red flag" warning for you.

Let's now turn to some interesting study findings that emerged during the Covid-19 lockdowns, when students and adults were tethered to their computers to complete school or work assignments. During this period, what were some of the reported adverse impacts on adults' activity routines and on their well-being—and what takeaways can we draw from these findings?

Let's first look at an interesting study completed in 2020 by a research team led by Professor Fei Qin from China, along with colleagues in the United States and Denmark. The team's motivation was to determine whether during the Covid-19 lockdowns adults were more likely to experience insufficient physical activity relative to the WHO-recommended standard and, if so, how it affected their well-being, including their moods.

To meet this objective, from January 25, 2020, through February 2, 2020—the period of Chinese New Year normally involving much face-to-face mingling among family and friends—the researchers recruited locked-down adults living in thirty-one provinces in China to complete an online physical activity and well-being survey. The geographic areas chosen for inclusion were based on the sampling plan of the sixth national physical fitness monitoring points system — drawing potential respondents from a wide area of China but excluding Taiwan, Hong Kong, and Macau, because they were not covered by the established fitness monitoring system.

Besides answering the typical questions about their age, gender, and education, participants were asked to complete the International Physical Activity Questionnaire (IPAQ), a key part of the survey. This questionnaire asks people to recall over the past week, the number of days per week and the number of minutes per day they engaged in sitting or vigorous physical activity, moderate physical activity, and walking. Participants were also asked to describe their moods during the lockdown by completing the Positive and Negative Affect Schedule (PANAS) survey items.

By the end of the data collection period, just over 12,000 adults completed the survey, ranging in age from 18 to 80 years. Most (69 percent) resided in rural China and self-identified as professionals (about 40 percent) or students (about 37 percent).

What were the major study findings of interest to us here? Not surprisingly, the amount of daily screen time far exceeded the expert-recommended two hours daily, with respondents saying they spent daily about 4 hours (or about 261 minutes) online for work or school activities. The age group citing the longest screen time (over 305 minutes a day) was that aged 20–29 years, and for all age groups, screen time increased as physical activity level declined.

As for physical activity during the Covid-19 lockdown, during the initial phase, nearly 60 percent of the respondents reported insufficient physical activity—more than twice WHO's "insufficient" physical activity prevalence rate of 27.5 percent. As expected, the lockdown adversely impacted Chinese citizens' activity level health—and negatively impacted their moods. In terms of mood, the adults pursuing vigorous physical activity even during the lockdown periods had significantly better emotional states, as reflected in higher positive affect scores. These physically active adults also spent significantly less time on their digital devices than those practicing lighter physical activity. The respondents who adopted a sedentary lifestyle during the lockdowns—marked by inadequate physical activity and lots of sitting—exhibited very poor emotional states, marked by elevated levels of negative mood and depression.

Given these findings, what are the key takeaways? The research team concluded that during the Covid-19 lockdowns, far too many Chinese adults routinely practiced insufficient physical activity—resulting in their being prone to over-use of screen time and negative moods. Because of the importance of physical activity in normative times or in high-stress periods, the researchers suggested that promotional campaigns by government need to emphasize how home-based walking and running regimens—a natural and generally permitted form of mindful untethering or digital detoxing even during extended or repeat lockdown periods—can help citizens safeguard their physical and mental well-being in both the short- and the long-term.

18. What are cyberbullying and cyberharassment? What should you do if you're a target?

While cyberbullying (also called "cyberharassment") and cyberstalking (called "criminal harassment" in Canada) are forms of psychological and behavioral abuses occurring in the virtual world, these abuses can also occur on land.

These online abuses typically cause various degrees of harm to targets, including elevating their anxiety and depression levels in the short term—and if persistent, often leading to suicide ideation or actual attempts by the victims. Both cyberbullying and cyberstalking place in the broader land-based category of "bullying," whereby victims cannot easily defend themselves against unwanted behaviors by their bullies or stalkers. Mental health experts warn that with so many teens highly engaged in social media, online abuses reported to close friends and law enforcement have increased significantly in recent years.

Cyberbullying is harassing someone online by sending a series of threatening emails or text messages. According to recent estimates, about 85 percent of girls and women globally have experienced it. Three defining characteristics for cyberbullying include a bully's: (1) intending to cause harm to another person—most often mentally; (2) repeating the harmful acts—though unwanted and perhaps even verbalized by the victim; and (3) imposing a power imbalance—with the bully trying to establish or maintain mental control over the victim.

Cyberstalking involves a stalker's using the internet to launch a targeted, often lengthy campaign against someone with the intent of causing *extreme* fear, distress, or alarm in the victim. In more severe cases, the stalker tries to mentally control the victim by threatening to injure or cause death to the victim, to the victim's friends or family members, or to the victim's pets or coworkers. A common trigger for stalkers to issue these kinds of heinous threats is if the victim says that he/she is leaving an existing relationship. It is also common for victims in the more advanced cases to experience both virtual and land-based bullying. These "hybrid" hostile acts can include: sending repeated and unwanted messages to the target; posting false or hostile information online about the victim; using social media sites to harass the victim; subscribing to online services or products in the victim's name; hacking the victim's personal accounts to maintain power and control; impersonating the victim online by engaging in identity theft; sending the victim files containing malware; and recruiting others to help threaten the victim.

Because of the dire consequences to victims of these abuses, a number of laws have been passed in various countries to deter such behaviors—with California, for example, passing the first land-based stalking law in the United States in 1991. There has also been considerable movement more recently to prevent online abuses, particularly those targeting minors. For example, in 2008, the US Congress passed the Protecting Children in the 21st Century legislation to address cyberbullying, and by 2011, at least forty-four US states had legislation in place to address school bullying, per se. Currently, there is renewed activism by parents who have lost their children to social media abuses to push the US government to pass the Kids Online Safety Act (KOSA), a bill introduced by Senators Blumenthal and Blackburn in February 2022 and reintroduced in May 2023.

Court cases involving serious virtually based abuse cases targeting teens have been reported by the media worldwide to help educate teens about the dangers existing online. One such case involved an anonymous perpetrator who cyberbullied and cyberstalked for two years a Canadian teen named Amanda Todd. Her highly distressing plight came into full display in 2012 after she posted a video on *YouTube* with flash cards and this message, "I've decided to tell you about my never ending story." In her video, Amanda shared with the world her trauma of being abused, bullied, harassed, and stalked online by some unidentified adult male in cyberspace, who threatened to tell her parents, friends, and school authorities if she refused to send him sexually revealing poses of herself. She said that she tried to cope with this very stressful situation by taking drugs, drinking alcohol, and mutilating parts of her body, but because this man's unrelenting abuse continued, she eventually died by suicide to avoid further pain or humiliation.

In January 2014, a 35-year-old Dutch man named Aydin Coban was identified and charged in the Netherlands for his ongoing virtual abuse campaigns against female teens globally—including Amanda's. His criminal charges were many and included online extortion, internet luring, cyberstalking, cyberharassment, and child pornography. Though it took almost a decade for Amanda's case to go to trial in Canada, the British Columbia judge recently hearing her case branded her perpetrator Coban as an "Internet sextortionist," sanctioning him to an unprecedented thirteen years in Canadian prison—once he finishes his prison term in the Netherlands.

School districts in the United States and elsewhere also have increasingly developed policies on bullying and cyberbullying to address the seriousness of the problem and to delineate sanctions for those engaging in such behaviors. These policies broadly prohibit the use of the school's internet system for inappropriate communications among peers. These policies also make it clear that there is a limited expectation of privacy when using technology on school premises, for such abuses will not be tolerated and are monitored. While there has been considerable controversy as to what authority schools have in the regulation of abusive student behavior occurring outside the school system, districts have nonetheless developed policies holding students accountable for their online behavior even when not on school premises.

Schools have also designed and implemented educational programs to prevent cyber abuses. For example, US curriculum-based programs are now widely used, including the iSAFE Internet Safety Program, the Cyber Bullying: A Prevention Curriculum, and the Let's Fight It Together: What We All Can Do to Prevent Cyber Bullying. These include videos on the types of cyber abuse and scripted lessons to help students have conversations about key issues and adopt remedies so they can better protect themselves. Sometimes counseling is provided for the abusers and/or the victims, and in the more severe abuse cases, the authorities are brought in to investigate.

How can teens protect themselves beyond these school abuse policies and educational programs? Here are some pointers shared by mental health experts to help you stay safe online: (1) do *not* share your personal information in public spaces via public networks or give your personal information to strangers online, including in emails or on social media sites; (2) do *not* use your real name as your user ID but instead use a gender- and age-neutral online moniker; (3) avoid meeting online acquaintances on land, and if you choose to meet someone not in your trust circle, do so in a public place and take a friend along; (4) make sure that your Internet Service Provider (ISP) has an acceptable use policy prohibiting cyber abuse—and file a complaint with the ISP if you experience offensive behaviors that violate their policy. If the ISP fails to act immediately, switch to a more responsive provider; and (5) if an online situation becomes extremely hostile or threatening, immediately log off and consider notifying school or legal authorities.

19. What user safety features are built into social media and messaging apps?

There is a growing sentiment globally that given the propensity of teens to be highly engaged in social media, society has allowed them to essentially enter "the cab of a dangerous cyber machine" and then let platforms like *TikTok*, *Twitter* (now *X*), and *Facebook* "take control of the wheel." That is why in concerned jurisdictions like the United States, Canada, and the UK, government hearings are taking place to ascertain the degree of risk built into social media and messaging apps so that governments can not only curb it but make platforms accountable.

Mental health experts have also argued that these platforms have zero incentive to enforce the cab entry age of thirteen where such jurisdictional restrictions exist. On the contrary, these companies seem incentivized through their algorithms to do whatever they can to "hook" their teen consumers to routinely and frequently engage in the platform for financial gain by enticing advertisers to enlist.

For this reason, in jurisdictions like the United States, governments are considering raising the cab entry age to sixteen so that users can better understand the lack of safety features built into social media and messaging apps. The bill is a proposed update to the Children's Online Privacy Protection Act (COPPA), a US law passed in 1998 prohibiting internet companies from collecting Personally Identifiable Information (PII) from anyone younger than thirteen without parental consent. If passed, this Act would be known as COPPA 2.0.

Given this reality, other jurisdictions like the European Union have made considerable progress in challenging the business model of social media companies. In fact, the EU's landmark privacy legislation passed in 2018, known as the General Data Protection Regulation (GDPR), has created stronger privacy rights for users. It has also created stronger obligations and guardrails for social media companies around the collection, retention, and management of users' personally identifiable information. In January 2023, EU regulators further buckled down on these companies by issuing large penalties for violations of key provisions in the GDPR. For example, Meta's *Facebook* found itself facing a $562 million privacy invasion fine, with EU regulators ruling that one of the components in its business model was illegal in that jurisdiction because of its "predatory" online business practices.

Evidence also continues to mount that for social media apps on smartphones, the harms to teen users can easily outweigh the benefits of their being connected. While social media platforms can provide teens struggling to form friendships in the land-based world a chance to connect with peers sharing common interests in the virtual world, mental health experts argue that social media feeds can expose users to cyberbullying and cyberstalking. Also, over-use of social media by teens, particularly at night, can rob them of much-needed REM sleep, curtail their concentration at school, and erode their self-esteem.

What's particularly alarming, affirm mental health experts, is that much of this harm occurs during social media users' life stages when the brain is especially vulnerable to changes. For example, in 2023, neuroscience researchers at the University of North Carolina found that in a series of brain scans on young people—by age twelve, "habitual" social media users already developed a hypersensitivity to peer feedback that would stay with them for life. By definition, habitual users check their social media feeds fifteen or more times a day, moderate users check theirs between one and fourteen times a day, and non-habitual users check theirs less than once a day. This study finding underscores a reality that the big tech companies are cognizant of but choose to deny: That the harms experienced by habitual social media users in the short term can make them susceptible to SNS addiction over the longer term.

In what ways are social media platforms addictive? In 2020, a Canadian psychiatric team led by Dr. Abi-Jaoude answered this question by positing that both social media and online gaming platforms have been designed in highly sophisticated ways using behavioral psychology, neuroscience, and Artificial Intelligence (AI) to promote *intense* user engagement. In particular, behavioral reinforcement techniques are employed to have users remain engaged for long periods of time and to return for more engagement, possibly leading to addiction to the platform. Again, the more users engage on the platform, the greater the opportunity for social media and online gaming companies to generate profits from targeted advertising. It is for this reason that advertisers are keenly interested in knowing the number of documented "heavy users" the platform has before committing advertising dollars to it!

So are there any guard rails built into SNSs to protect users? Apparently not! Witness the 2021 testimony of *Facebook* whistle-blower Frances Haugen, who told US Congress that her former employer ignored internal research findings that habitual engagement in *Instagram* (which *Meta* owns along with *Facebook*) caused 33 percent of teen females to feel worse about themselves and their bodies after routinely engaging on the platform. Yet, affirmed Haugen, company executives carried on with their profit-making and their advertising-centric business plans without disclosing this finding.

Add to this evidence the fact that *Twitter's* former head of IT security Peiter Zatko (aka "Mudge") told the US Justice Department during a 2022 hearing that a number of his company's business policies and actions unquestionably put consumers in harm's way. He detailed extensive legal violations, including *Twitter's* making misleading statements to users about how their personal information, provided for platform access, would be used. He said that the company acted with "negligence and even complicity" toward conscious efforts made by foreign governments (like China) to infiltrate the SNS platform for their own financial gain, placing young users at additional risk.

20. What is hate speech, and how can you protect yourself from it online?

Before defining what hate speech is and how we online users can protect ourselves from it, let's look at how prevalent it is thought to be. According to Emily Laidlaw, a Canada Research Chair in Cybersecurity Law and a professor at the University of Calgary, a recent 2022 Abacus Data poll commissioned by the Canadian Race Relations Foundation found that a remarkable one in five Canadians said that they experienced online hate, harassment, or violence. Women, 2SLGBTQ+ individuals, online users living in racialized communities, Jews, Muslims, and teens were especially vulnerable to being targeted.

Furthermore, according to recent Statscan data, hate crimes continue to mount year after year in both land-based and online environments. For example, the number of hate crimes reported by the Canadian and military police grew by 27 percent to 3,360 in 2021 from 2,646 incidents reported in 2020. The primary targets were those in the LGBTQ, Muslim, and Jewish communities. What's alarming is that about half of these hate crimes involved violent acts like assault, harassment, and uttering threats, and much of this hate rhetoric appears to be generated by individuals identifying with the far right politically in North America and elsewhere. Also, there seems to be a significant rise in those who feel emboldened to take their hate speech from an anonymous online space to an in-person, land-based space. Notably, in 2023 with the advent of the Israeli-Hamas war, hate crimes in the United States against Jews rose by a whopping 400 percent within one month.

But what exactly is hate speech and how can it be managed? First, it is important to recognize that hate speech laws where they do exist are not only perplexing and difficult to manage but that there exists quite a degree of variability in interpretation in some jurisdictions, compared to others. In China, North Korea, and Russia, for example, restrictions regarding free speech are really quite pronounced. In more open jurisdictions valuing Free Speech—such as Canada and the United States, laws exist to try to prevent individuals from abusing their Free Speech privileges by placing others at risk of harm by uttering hate propaganda or hate speech. But what exactly is "hate speech"?

In Canada, for example, legal authorities say that for a message to be deemed as "hate propaganda" or "hate speech" under Canada's Criminal Code, the message has to be made publicly, and it must target one of five identifiable protected groups based on race, color, religion, ethnic origin, or sexual orientation. Authorities in this jurisdiction must determine whether someone online or on land is attempting to incite disdain or hatred toward a particular protected group and to gather convincing evidence before charging the perpetrator(s) under the Criminal Code.

Now let's turn to the United States, where under the First Amendment to the Constitution, offensive online content and hate speech have the same protections as any other form of land-based speech. Some experts would even posit that hate organizations in the United States are relatively protected when they launch their hate messages online. Why? Because the same First Amendment protections apply to *all* US citizens—including social media influencers like Kanye West (aka Ye), who in 2022 voiced his anti-Semitic tirades on social media, causing companies like German sportswear manufacturer *Adidas* to end its lucrative partnership with the rapper in order to safeguard their brand.

So is there any effective way for online citizens to control hate speech, particularly if they live in a less restrictive area like the United States? Because the First Amendment guarantees freedom of speech broadly, at the present time, even the US government is quite limited in its ability to regulate online hate speech through its existing civil and criminal laws. So there currently is a movement on there to make the social media platforms more accountable for monitoring and removing hate speech once a complaint by an online user has been received. However, even this attempt at accountability has proven difficult for platform censors, given that the principle underlying online free speech is the promotion of "a marketplace of ideas," in which distasteful or offensive speech is answered "by more speech." Within this so-called "marketplace of ideas," online citizens are encouraged to work through posted beliefs and ideals that best resonate with them and avoid SNSs having content that does not resonate well.

In other words, once "hate speech" aimed at a particular gender, sexual orientation, or religion is displayed publicly in an online forum—such as on social media, it can then be responded to by other users' arguments revealing its falsity and offensiveness and, through a series of counter-postings, online users can advocate for more positive and enlightened values.

In 2023, it is important to note that the US Supreme Court is reconsidering key tenets of online speech to give the social media networks more accountability. For years, the giant social media networks *Facebook*, *Twitter*, and *Instagram* have operated under two crucial tenets: (1) That social media platforms through their usage policies have the power to decide what content to keep online and what to take down, and (2) that the websites *cannot* be held legally responsible for most of what users post online. For these two reasons, social media platforms have viewed themselves as being shielded from lawsuits over libelous speech, extremist content, and real-world harms linked to their platforms.

Given this present-day dilemma, the US Supreme Court is poised to reconsider those two rules, potentially leading to the most significant reset of the doctrines governing online speech since the courts decided to apply few regulations to the internet in the 1990s. The two current Supreme Court cases *Gonzalez v. Google* and *Twitter v. Taamneh* specifically challenge Section 230 of the Communications Decency Act (CDA), which holds newspapers and other print media liable when violating this section of the Act, especially when offensive comments are made in print. The key tenet that the Supreme Court will need to address is this: Why make print media accountable, yet protect social media platforms from lawsuits when their online users post offensive remarks or when the platform censors decide to take down posts that they deem to be offensive and against the platform's policies?

The bottom line is this: It looks as though we will have to wait to see what the outcomes of these two Supreme Court challenges (and others elsewhere) are as the growing global battle over how to best handle harmful speech online and on land remains a yet unsolved mystery for governments, citizens, and the social media platforms.

Protecting Your Money and Identity Online

21. What laws exist in the United States to safeguard your finances, identity, and medical records online?

Where you live in the world will determine the effectiveness of the privacy protection laws existing there to safeguard your personally identifiable information (PII), while online. PII generally pertains to your finances (such as your bank account numbers and balances), your identity data (such as your social security number or driver's license number), and your medical records (such as diagnosed illnesses you are being medically treated for by a medical health practitioner). Some privacy laws apply to businesses collecting and retaining clients' and employees' PII, while other laws apply strictly to federal branches of government, like banking.

How effectively these privacy laws protect your PII depends on the severity of sanctions imposed when the laws are violated and on the funding amounts allocated by government to the regulators' or privacy watchdogs' activities. These regulators typically have titles like "Office of the Privacy Commissioner (OPC)" and are affiliated, say, with federal or state/provincial levels in the United States and Canada.

In numerous polls taken over the last thirty years—whether completed in the United States, Britain, or Canada, citizens living in these democratic jurisdictions have expressed strong concerns about their governments' providing adequate protections for their PII, whether on land or online. These polls have underscored that privacy protection has long been considered a fundamental right for citizens, covered by some form of Charter of Rights and Freedoms.

Let's take a closer look now at various laws protecting citizen's online PII. In the United States, there is no single data protection regulation. Rather, hundreds of laws exist at the federal and state levels. At the federal level, the Federal Trade Commission Act (FTCA) broadly empowers the Federal Trade Commission

(FTC) to not only protect consumers against unfair or deceptive data collection and dissemination practices but to enforce federal privacy and data protection regulations. According to the FTC, "deceptive practices" include a company's failure to provide adequate Security, Privacy, and Trust (PST) to employees' and clients' PII. In addition, the company cannot use the data collected and maintained to engage in deceptive marketing or advertising means. Other federal statutes address particular societal sectors, such as financial services, health care, education, and telecommunications.

US Federal laws safeguarding PII are extensive, including these five: (1) The Gramm Leach Bliley Act (GLBA), governing protections of consumers' PII by banks, insurance companies, and financial services companies; (2) The Fair Credit Reporting Act (FCRA), restricting the use of information dealing with citizens' credit scores and standing; (3) The Health Information Portability and Accountability Act (HIPPA) protecting information held by medical entities regarding patients' health status or treatments; (4) The Family Education and Privacy Act (FERPA), giving students the right to revise their student records for accuracy, while prohibiting the disclosure of this information to third parties without the students' or their parents' consent; and (5) The Children's Online Privacy Protection Act (COPPA) prohibits the online collection of any PII from minors under the age of thirteen or without their parental consent.

At the US state level, privacy protections vary, with some states having quite comprehensive protections, ranging from safeguarding citizens' library records to keeping homeowners' properties free from drone surveillance.

In the UK, the key federal data protection law is the 2018 General Data Protection Regulation (GDPR), serving as a model piece of legislation not only because of its "teeth" in protecting citizens' online PII, but because it is very well funded. In fact, the GDPR authorizes an annual registration fee to be paid by *every* business that handles employees' and clients' PII. This enhanced funding model allows Britain's Information Commissioner's Office (BICO) to showcase its effectiveness both as a regulator when employee or consumer complaints are filed and when policies need to be developed for rapid responses by businesses to protect PII after network data breaches occur (such as present-day ransomware attacks).

In Canada, the OPC is the federal regulator for online privacy protections, but unlike the UK, the OPC is "a poor sister." The OPC gets just under 50 cents per capita annually for enforcing Canada's federal privacy law, known as the Personal Information Protection and Electronic Documents Act (PIPEDA). If the Act is violated by businesses, the OPC investigates and can make a recommendation to the Attorney General's Office (AGO) to levy sanctions.

Interestingly, in these three jurisdictions, the business sector often brought to bear for abusing the privacy protections of citizens is social media companies. For example, in 2023, *Meta* (owning *Facebook, Instagram, Messenger,* and *WhatsApp*) suffered a major defeat after EU regulators found that its PII data collection method and rampant use of "targeted ads" failed to be consistent with GDPR key provisions. As a result, *Meta* was not only required to pay a huge fine of $558 million but was required to make changes to their business model to bring it in line with the GDPR provisions. If *Meta* failed to comply in a timely fashion, they would face further sanctions.

22. Is it safe to use public wi-fi?

Is it safe to use public wi-fi at an airport or a coffee shop? No, affirm IT security experts, particularly if you are planning to open or transfer files containing confidential information (like your bank account number and password). Though many of us are probably tempted to use "open" public wi-fi networks at airports or hotels to get some work done, connect with friends, or play online games to relieve boredom, the cautionary note here is that you are risking the Privacy, Security, and Trust (PST) of your PII if you do so!

In fact malinclined hackers may be lurking on this open network looking for potential victims in order to steal their PII. Four common hack attacks known to occur in this not-secure environment include: (1) *Man-in-the-Middle Attacks,* whereby a hacker places himself/herself between you and your connection to public wi-fi—thus gaining access to all that you are doing on your digital device like accessing your bank account; (2) *Evil Twin Attacks,* whereby a hacker creates a fake wi-fi account and makes it look authentic—so if you are at an airport trying to log onto an assumed "safe open" network, you may find two names looking very similar (like AirportNetwork1 and AirportNetwork12); likely one of these is an "evil twin," allowing the hacker to gain full access to your information; (3) *Malware-Infected Networks,* whereby a hacker or some previous connector to the network deposits malware into the open network that could easily spread to other devices connected to it—including yours; and (4) *Session Hijacking,* whereby a hacker replicates all of the data on your device and then pretends to be you—having full control of your device and all the accounts on it, thus committing identity theft.

So how can you keep your PII safe while in hotels or airports? Answer: Avoid open networks! Here are five other tips offered by IT security experts: (1) Use a VPN (Virtual Private Network), obtainable for free or for a fee, to encrypt all of your data—making it inaccessible to hackers; (2) use a password manager, an encrypted space that safely stores your passwords until you need to use one; (3) do not access or log into your highly confidential accounts while in public spaces; (4) do not click on random links or pop-ups that may appear on your device; and (5) enable two-factor authentication to prevent loss of data—and if you do get an alert that someone has suspiciously logged onto your device (but not you), change your password immediately and run an anti-virus scan.

23. What is phishing, and how can you spot a fake email or text message?

Phishing, or spear-phishing, is an attempted form of identity theft, whereby a cyber fraudster uses an authentic-looking email from your company's executives, your school's administrator, or some other "trusted" company to trick you into disclosing sensitive personal information—such as your credit card number or your bank account codes.

What the cyber fraudster is hoping is that you will fall for his/her fake email scheme. While IT departments try to educate students and employees about the dangers of clicking on URLs in unexpected and *likely untrustworthy* emails, inevitably the warned one ignores the training and clicks on it anyway— unleashing onto the network some harmful malware or sharing his/her PII that can be used to steal one's identity.

So how common is phishing? In 2022, IT security experts at *Mimecast* (a British-American firm), say there were an estimated 225 million spear-phishing attempts reported by companies—a whopping 61 percent increase over those reported in 2021! A significant 90 percent of the companies said that the negative consequences of successful phishing exploits included online account compromises, data breaches targeting clients and employees, and costly data freezes because of ransomware attacks—whereby the bad guys demand a ransom for the alleged exchange of a "decryptor key" to unlock frozen data. IBM IT security experts have also confirmed that in 2022, phishing was the most costly attack vector used by cyber criminals to invade companies' networks—costing an estimated $4.91 million worth of damages with each hit.

Microsoft IT security experts confirm that there are at least six "garden varieties" of dangerous phishing emails/texts/phone calls to be on the lookout for, including these: (1) *Email*, the most common type, occurs when bad actors use a wide-net approach by employing phony hyperlinks to masquerade as some well-known account provider (like *Google*) to entice email receivers to share their PII; (2) *Malware* occurs when bad actors implant it into an email disguised as a trustworthy attachment (like a bank statement), but once the attachment is opened by the receiver, the entire network can become negatively affected; (3) *Spear phishing,* a form of highly customized email and content typically able to bypass network security measures in place, because it targets those with authorized high-level network access (such as employees in Finance) so that the bad guys can extort money; (4) *Whaling,* potentially very lucrative, occurs when the bad actors target a "big fish" like a business executive or a celebrity in the hopes that they can successfully steal that user's login credentials or other sensitive personal information; (5) *Smishing* (a combo of "SMS" and "phishing") occurs when bad actors send text messages looking as though they come from legitimate sources (like *FedEx*) in an effort to lure receivers into responding quickly—often by sending money; and (6) *Vishing* (a combo of VoIP and phishing), a form of "social engineering," occurs when bad actors use fraudulent call centers to lure receivers into providing their personal information (such as credit card numbers) over the phone or convincing them to install an app onto their devices that is actually malware.

How might you protect yourself from the dangers of phishing? Here are five useful tips and "red flags" generally shared by IT security experts: (1) Don't trust the email source on the first read but instead check the sender's IP address before opening the email or responding—as the display name could be a fake; (2) don't trust the content if an email has lots of spelling errors and/or poor grammar, because it likely is phishing; (3) don't trust the sender if the salutation of an email starts with something vague like, "Dear Valued Customer"; (4) don't trust the sender if an email does not provide contact information, because it likely is phishing; and (5) don't trust the sender if there is a threatening statement in the email header like, "Your account has been frozen."

24. What is the difference between phishing and spamming?

Phishing is an email, text message, or phone call customized in some way so that the receiver is lured into sharing PII—like credit card numbers—that can be used by the bad guys for identity theft. Spam, on the other hand, is not customized but involves a much larger net of potentially gullible victims, who receive unsolicited, unwanted, and impersonal emails asking for personal information or to make a purchase.

Generally, spam has these three characteristics differentiating it from phishing: (1) The receiver's personal identity is irrelevant, because the email sent is applicable to many other receivers; (2) the receiver has not given explicit consent for the email, and (3) the email appears to give a "disproportionate benefit" to the sender rather than to the receiver.

Simply put, spam is, for the most part, a nuisance to email receivers, for it wastes our time. However, law enforcement experts warn that spam may contain content that is not only offensive but likely criminally motivated; for example, it may be marketing child pornography. Furthermore, spam is a nuisance to organizations, for it negatively impacts employees' productivity. While most businesses today employ spam filters to reduce the likelihood of spam receipt, some of the spam messages do slip through the system.

Why are humans so gullible that spammers occasionally successfully bait unsuspecting "fish"? Answer: Because spammers, like most of us, are honing their tech skills and getting better at conning us. If as an individual, you've been scammed at least once and still feel distressed about it, you are not alone. In 2022, the Canadian Anti-Fraud Centre, for example, said that Canadian residents lost at least $530 million to scammers who are becoming much more tech-savvy and better at their social engineering capabilities.

Why do victims fall for scams even though they may detect some "red flags" in the spammer's marketing pitch? Jeff Hancock, a communications professor at Stanford University, says it is because *homo sapiens* are inherently gullible and overly trusting creatures. Because humans are "wired" to take people at face value and to believe that what they say is true, we tend to act on our sometimes false perceptions. He refers to it as "the truth bias," affirming that this is how in an evolutionary sense, we humans have been able to build relationships, conduct business, and manage our daily lives.

Professor Hancock offers these four pointers to help ward off our gullible impulses: (1) If your initial perception is that something sounds "too good to be true," it likely is; (2) if the scammer wants you to act immediately because there is an urgency to get the act done *now*, take a step back and forego acting impulsively; (3) if you are hesitant about discussing this so-called "special opportunity" with other trusted friends, your instincts are telling you that likely something is wrong; and (4) if you are phoned or contacted online with remarkable propositions from strangers, do not engage in dialogue with them but disconnect politely to keep yourself safe.

25. What should you do if you think you've been the victim of online fraud?

Online fraud occurs when someone tries to steal funds or other valuable information from you using devious and illegal means. Ransomware attacks are present-day examples of online fraud, such that your data becomes locked (or encrypted) by hackers until you pay a ransom to allegedly get a decryption key to unfreeze your data.

By definition, "online fraud" encompasses a wide range of criminal activities occurring in virtual space—aptly called cybercrimes—that bring various degrees of harm to targets if successfully executed. These online activities include attempts to steal intellectual property rights (IPR), PII, trade secrets, or credit card information. Because the harms produced by online fraud can be extensive, in the United States, the Internet Fraud Complaint Center (IFCC), a partnership between the FBI and the National White Collar Crime Center (NW3C), was created to help mitigate these harms (now called the Internet Crime Complaint Center, or IC3). Other jurisdictions have created similar kinds of government internet crime reporting centers, such as the Canadian Anti-Fraud Centre.

So, how do online fraudsters successfully execute their missions? Short answer: They are good at lying convincingly, even virtually. Their untruthful behavior technically places in the broader category of "social engineering," whereby the perpetrator brazenly attempts to dupe naive or overly-trusting individuals. More often than not, the fraudster will use skillful deception to manipulate individuals into divulging confidential or personal information that may be used for various kinds of fraudulent purposes, including identity theft.

In a modern-day real-life case in point, Guo Wengui, a 54-year-old man long sought by the Chinese government on corruption grounds, has strong connections with other wealthy business people, even in North America. He, in fact, supposedly cultivated close links to former President Trump's administration to advance his own financial goals. In 2023, he was arrested by US authorities on charges that he orchestrated a $1 billion online fraud conspiracy. He and his financier colleague Kin Ming Je now face an indictment in US federal court on multiple criminal charges—including wire, securities, and bank fraud. US prosecutors say that the indictment stems from a complex scheme in which the pair *successfully lied* to hundreds of thousands of online followers in the United States and elsewhere before misappropriating hundreds of millions of dollars from their victims. Not only did this pair of fraudsters "line their pockets" with the stolen money, but they bought a 50,000 sq ft mansion, a $3.5 million Ferrari, and a $37 million luxury yacht. If the pair is found guilty of all of these charges, they face more than 100 years in prison.

If this pair of cybercriminals could dupe business-savvy professionals by deploying their well-honed social engineering capabilities, what does that say about "netizens" who fear that they may become naive victims of online fraud? Is their fear justified, given the prevalence of reported cases in North America? According to the Canadian Better Business Bureau (BBB), the percentage of Canadians who reported losing money after being targeted by an online scam increased to 46.9 percent in 2022 from 45.1 percent in 2021, so, yes, this fear does seem justified.

If you think you have been the victim of online fraud, report your incident to your jurisdiction's equivalent of the BBB or the Canadian Anti-Fraud Centre online tracking system to help protect others. There is no shame in dealing with the fraud aftermath, since anyone of any age who is on social media or has a mobile phone can become an online fraud victim. According to the BBB, people of different ages are susceptible to particular kinds of online and mobile phone scams. Those 65 and older, for example, are more likely to lose money when contacted by phone, those aged 35–44 are more likely to be targeted through social media, and those aged 25–44 are more likely to become victims when contacted through text messages. Also, affirms the BBB, Canadian women (about 64 percent) have reported being the victim of online scams, compared to men (about 37 percent), although the median scam loss reported by men ($453) was almost double that reported by women ($249).

Finally, the BBB shares these four pointers to help safeguard yourself: (1) Watch out for "red flags" online like "cash-only" deals, high "up-front" payments, "handshake" deals without a contract, and unsolicited services like "free" on-site home inspections; (2) protect yourself by not believing everything you see or read online, for even though a website or an email may look official on quick glance, there is no guarantee that it is—for even mobile phone caller IDs can be realistically faked; (3) never share your PII—like your social security number or driver's license number—with someone who has contacted you online or by phone and whose action was unsolicited by you; and (4) use secure, *traceable* transactions when making payments online for goods and services—because though transactions made through your secure online bank account can be traced, pre-paid gift cards bought online cannot be.

26. How can you protect yourself from becoming a victim of online identity theft?

"Identity theft" is the malicious stealing and consequent misuse of someone else's identity by gaining illegal access to their PII—including their social security numbers, bank account numbers, driver's license numbers, and network passwords. Without question, the internet enables the more traditional land-based identity theft criminals to gain access to many more targets in multiple jurisdictions without leaving home.

IT security experts have warned that because far too many online users freely share their PII with others in the virtual world—including strangers, they can easily become identity theft victims. Also, if a company's or a school district's network has been the target of a hack attack, chances are the PII of the company's clients/employees or the school's staff/students has fallen into the hands of cybercriminals. Cybercriminals, of course, will potentially use that PII to benefit themselves financially. The stolen PII may even be sold to other cybercriminals lurking in the depths of the World Wide Web known as the "Dark Web." This is where digital-savvy child pornographers, weapons dealers, and drug cartels reside and benefit greatly from their illegal business transactions.

How do IT security experts say that you can protect yourself against identity theft? First, you need to become educated about the various forms of internet fraud in existence in your particular jurisdiction—such as the circulating phishing scams and the online fraud schemes. One easy way to do this is to routinely review the "alerts" posted on your Cybercrime Complaint Center's website. For example, if you reside in the United States, you would consult the Internet Crime Complaint Center (IC3). Second, you should regularly review the protection "tips" located on that website—because the practical tips cited are routinely updated for particular kinds of reported scams or frauds.

Here are five broad-based tips that Cybercrime Complaint Center experts often share with online users to help them reduce the likelihood of identity theft: (1) Refrain from opening links generated by suspicious email addresses; (2) verify as legitimate any websites claiming to be an official government website by contacting your relevant government office before sharing your PII; (3) confirm with your financial institution that any requested information regarding, say, a loan repayment is legitimate and was generated by them and not by some online scammer; (4) use tremendous caution when asked to input your PII or financial information onto a non-trustworthy website; and (5) look for spelling or grammatical errors on a so-called legitimate website, in email, or in text messages—for these are very likely "red flags" indicating you are being approached by an online scammer or fraudster.

Importantly, if you think have already been duped by a scammer, here are four additional tips that you should follow: (1) Notify immediately your Crime Complaint Center (like the IC3) by filing an incident complaint—to protect yourself and others; (2) notify immediately the online payment service used for the financial transaction(s) in question and ask them to stop or reverse the transaction(s), if it is feasible to do so; (3) keep all transaction information— including prepaid credit cards, banking records, and phone/text/email communications with the scammer—and promptly provide such to authorities, if and when requested to do so; (4) and monitor routinely your financial and credit card accounts for any suspicious fraudulent activity, and immediately notify your financial institution if any charges look amiss to you.

Finally, to help guard against identity theft, you might consider investing in specially designed software available on the consumer market, such as that provided by *Norton* or *McAfee*. In terms of the approximate cost for this kind of software protection, the *Norton Lifelock* product, for example, currently charges subscribers about $9 per month.

27. What is a data breach and how can you protect yourself after one has occurred?

Most democratic jurisdictions like the United States, Canada, Australia, and the UK have strong data breach notification and broad-based consumer protection laws when there is a Real Risk of Significant Harm (RRoSH) to victims after a network has been hacked by bad actors. These consumer protection laws exist because, as underscored in 2022 by Canadian journalist Joe Castaldo, in 52 percent of modern-day network hack attacks known as "ransomware," the bad actors not only encrypt the stolen data but threaten to post it in the bowels of the Dark Web.

These ransomware attacks have become quite commonplace in the United States, Canada, and elsewhere over the past few years. In September 2023, for example, the notorious Russian ransomware group called Lockbit threatened to leak internal data from The Weather Network's parent company onto the Dark Web after their cyber attack crippled operations of the Canadian company for several days. The hacker gang bragged that they had downloaded a lot of databases from the network, including codes to the company's digital servers—which they threatened to publish online if the ransom demanded was not quickly paid.

There is little question that the cost to society of data breaches like the one just described is enormous. In fact, it is estimated that by 2025, cybercrime globally is expected to cost $10.5 trillion annually, up from $3.5 trillion in 2015. As IT security experts are known to warn: No network is truly safe from hack attacks, so apply the security protections you have available and consider investing in more—for it's not a matter of if but when your network will be exploited. On a cautionary note, even the casinos in Las Vegas, notably big spenders on high-level security safeguards because they are keen to keep their networks safe from intruders, have recently been hacked. MGM Resorts International was, in fact, the target of a costly cyberattack that lasted ten days until September 20, 2023. Consequently, MGM management shut down all slot machines to prevent the hackers from forcibly paying out all their cash! Still, analysts estimate that the losses there cost MGM between $20 million and $40 million.

For this critical reason, jurisdictions around the globe have implemented consumer data protection laws in the event of a hack attack. The first such piece of US legislation was passed in 2003 in California and was called the California Security Breach Notification Act. This Act's passage was in response to a massive data breach at a California state agency when the names, addresses, and social security number of employees put them at Real Risk of Harm (resulting in such harms as workplace humiliation, job loss, reputation or relationship loss, financial loss, and property loss). Under this law, individuals affected by a network breach have to be notified *immediately* by the agency collecting, storing, or distributing individuals' PII so that these individuals can take remedial measures to safeguard their identities and reduce further harms. In 2008, California updated this law to include breaches involving online medical record and health insurance risks, and since then, the state has updated the law to require expedient notice of the breach to the US Attorney General.

Other US states quickly passed similar consumer protection legislation, and by 2012, breach notification laws existed in forty-six states. In 2015, President Obama passed legislation imposing a thirty-day deadline on agencies and enterprises for notifying likely victims following a network breach, as well as requiring the network owner to provide protective coverage to help mitigate potential harms, such as identity theft protection and credit monitoring for a stipulated period of time.

Various democracies globally have passed similar types of legislation to protect their online citizens from the aftermath of data breaches. In Canada, the relevant piece of legislation is known as PIPEDA (Personal Information Protection and Electronic Documents Act) and in the UK, it is the General Data Protection Regulation (GDPR). In all of these jurisdictions, PII is consistently defined as "information collected and stored in the system about individuals, where it is reasonably assumed that they can be identified using that piece of stolen information alone or in combination with other information."

Furthermore, agencies or businesses collecting and storing data on employees or clients must adhere to these four key principles in order to be legally compliant: (1) *Transparency*, such that they are required to clearly identify the purposes for which the PII is being collected at or before the time the information is collected; (2) *Lawful Basis for Processing*, such that they are required to collect PII by fair and lawful means (meaning that consent *cannot* be obtained from consumers or employees through deception, coercion, or misleading business practices); (3) *Purpose Limitation, Data Minimalization, and Proportionality*, such that they are required when collecting the PII to limit in type and in volume only that necessary to fulfill the business purposes transparently stated and not for other purposes any reasonable person would consider as "inappropriate" in the circumstances; and (4) *Retention*, such that they would keep the PII only for as long as necessary to fulfill the business/agency purposes for which it was identified, subject to a valid legal requirement.

Also, under these laws, employees and consumers are generally protected by four principles, including these: (1) They must be transparently informed about why their PII is being collected; (2) they can request corrections and/or deletions of inaccuracies or incompleteness of their PII; (3) they can withdraw their consent at any time, subject to legal or contractual restrictions, and with reasonable notice; and (4) they can not only withdraw consent to the use of their PII for marketing purposes but can file a complaint to the relevant Data Protection Authority (typically an OPC)—if noncompliance is perceived to have occurred.

Finally, you may be wondering how can you protect yourself if your employer or your school district has sent you a data breach notification letter that their network has been hacked? The best advice is to simply follow the mitigation strategies outlined in your letter. Common practices include telling you to immediately reset your network password, to engage in the credit monitoring protocol on offer, and to monitor any unauthorized charges made to your credit card or withdrawals made to your banking account. Importantly, *if any such illegal transactions are believed to have occurred, you should immediately notify your bank, the issuing credit card company, and the police.*

28. What is a ransom attack? How can you protect yourself, and what should you do if you become a target of a ransom attack?

Ransomware attacks "freeze" files by encrypting the data in the targeted network until such time as the demanded ransom is paid to the hacker gang that has exploited the network. The ransom is usually requested in cryptocurrency (like *Bitcoin*) so that tracing of the funds cannot easily occur. What's more, these bad actors tend to threaten to delete, disclose, or sell off the stolen data on the Dark Web—adding further pressure on victim organizations, government agencies, or school districts to quickly meet the bad actors' ransom demands.

Though the ransomware gangs may advise their targets that with timely ransom payments they will release a "decryption" key to unfreeze the stolen data, IT security experts warn that there is no guarantee that this outcome will actually occur! Furthermore, these experts caution that enterprises experiencing a ransomware attack should *not pay* the ransom demanded, for it not only encourages criminal behavior but there is a solid chance that the gang will launch another hack attack on the just hit network. Instead of paying the bad guys, companies should back up all of their data in the Cloud so that recovery can occur as quickly as possible following a known network breach.

What amounts of ransom have typically been demanded? While the amount has varied from one attack to another, often the amounts requested increase exponentially if the gangs know that the target is lucrative and has the means to pay large sums of currency. According to US law enforcement agencies, the notorious LockBit cybercriminals have demanded in the last two years at least $100 million in ransom payments from more than 1,000 victim enterprises in the United States, alone.

Also, IT security experts at the Canadian technology company Blackberry state on their current security blog that the Russian-based LockBit gang has been implicated in more cyber attacks in 2023 than any other ransomware gang operating in cyberspace. Interestingly, while LockBit's malware is designed to attack targeted networks in the United States, Canada, Europe, Asia, and Latin

America, newly minted LockBit 2.0 has been designed to "ignore" networks in the Commonwealth of Independent States and most Eastern Europe nations—except for Ukraine.

Nowadays, ransomware groups inhabiting the Dark Web continually change how they organize themselves. For example, one hacker group may "specialize" in a certain aspect of a ransomware attack—such as gaining initial access to a network, stealing data, demanding payment, or laundering payments. Another hacker group specializing in a different skill set might offer to become a partner with other gangs to successfully complete a massive hack attack. The "partner" groups would then share the "Spoils" once the ransom demanded has been paid. Each group, in effect, operates as an independent "Ransomware as a Service (RaaS)" consultant. This kind of outsourcing of a gang's skill set not only produces greater economic yields for the bad guys but makes them even harder to catch and be brought to justice for the horrific harms they cause, regardless of the jurisdiction in which the harms took place.

So what if your company's or school district's network has been hit by ransomware? Do you need to worry? As noted, employees, staff, or students who have been informed that they are likely part of a pool of PII currently "owned" by a ransomware gang should be vigilant. For your own protection against possible personal harms (like identity theft), you need to follow the guidelines given to you by your enterprise or school.

For example, in a recent Canadian ransomware attack occurring between January 16, 2023, and February 8, 2023, current and former employees at Canada's largest bookstore chain, *Indigo Books & Music Inc.*, had their social insurance numbers, financial details, and other PII leaked onto the Dark Web after a LockBit ransomware attack brought down the retailer's website. The good news is that the company was compliant with existing data protection legislation. The company's President told employees immediately that their personal information may have been acquired by an unauthorized third party and that as a means of protecting themselves, employees should consider contacting their local police, visiting the Canadian Anti-Fraud Centre for support, and reviewing the RCMP's Identity Theft and Identity Fraud Victim Assistance Guide for further steps. The President added that through *TransUnion of Canada, Inc.*, a consumer reporting agency, the company had arranged a two-year subscription to help employees monitor any critical changes to their credit scores. The subscription would also provide the monitoring of the surface Web (where we typically do our *Google* searches), the Deep Web, and the Dark Web for potentially exposed personal, identity, and financial information of employees as a means of alerting them early on about identity theft detection.

29. What is the Dark Web, and how is it different from the Deep Web?

We have discussed what ransomware is and how it is used by bad actors in cyber space for their own financial gain. We have also mentioned that ransomware-attacked businesses may tell their staff and/or clients that they will monitor the surface World Wide Web, the Deep Web, and the Dark Web to help identify victims at particular risk for identity theft.

But what is the difference between the Deep Web and the Dark Web? According to IT security experts, the Dark Web is where ransomware gangs, drug cartels, and child pornographers like to "do business." The Dark Web is essentially a hidden network of websites requiring special tools like the Tor router to gain access. The appeal of the Dark Web is that users with these special tools can enter here and remain anonymous—allowing them to exchange sensitive information with other like-minded individuals without commonly fearing retaliation by law enforcement.

That said, the World Wide Web should be viewed as being divided into several zones. The "surface zone" is the internet most online users are familiar with, where they can communicate with friends on social media websites, do searches on *Google*, and buy things online. The Deep Web and the Dark Web zones, on the other hand, are not accessible through search engines. Users wanting to engage in these two zones need special access privileges to enter.

Unlike the Dark Web, the Deep Web zone is not intrinsically malinclined or maldesigned. In fact, companies commonly communicate with their own employees through this zone, essentially an Intranet. In the Deep Web, for example, a company's privileged documents can be easily shared with work colleagues, and it is here that employees can search database entries while on their company's designated website.

To enter the Dark Web zone, as noted, visitors need the Tor router. To reach a desired Dark Web website but remain at relatively low risk for detection, a user's computer, by design, takes a random path to its destination, bouncing around a number of encrypted connections that seamlessly mask one's location and one's identity. But the bad guys are not the only inhabitants on the Dark Web. Nowadays, very tech-savvy law enforcement agents are actively using Tor to gain access to this zone in an effort to bring the bad guys to justice, often with the cooperation of agents across jurisdictions globally.

Privacy, Piracy, and Fake News Online

30. What are cookies, and how do websites use them?

According to the *Webster's New World Hacker Dictionary*, contrary to what you and others may think, cookies are not in themselves a security risk to users. Cookies are simply small bits of data commonly transmitted from a Web server to a Web browser, and they can be entirely processed client-side. The browser stores the message in a text file, and each time the browser requests from the server a particular Web page, the message is sent back to the server.

One of the most prevalent uses for cookies is to personalize any given Website for online users. So when users enter a Website, they may be asked to complete forms indicating their names or some other personally identifiable information (PII). Rather than experiencing some generic welcome page on their return to the Website, users are greeted with a more customized page that includes their identifiers stored in the cookies.

In today's privacy-focused society, there has been some controversy surrounding cookies. For example, cookies can be accessed, read, and used by malicious Websites unintentionally visited by innocent online users. In fact, cookie information can be used to gather intelligence on the online user and later be employed by the bad actors against the user. It is for this reason that online users are typically warned about the use of cookies and may be asked for their consent to continue on that particular Website.

You may, in fact, see a "cookie use" warning similar to this: This Website uses cookies to personalize our content and ads, to provide social media features, and to analyze our traffic—all with the intent of improving your experience as a user. We also share information about your use of our Website with our social media, advertising, and data analytics partners. They may combine our information with other information that you've provided to them, or that they've collected from your use of their services, for their own business purposes.

In jurisdictions with privacy protection laws, companies must notify online users why their PII is being collected and for what business purposes. So, it is quite common for a company's "cookie policy page" to display this important privacy protection information. Also, to remain compliant with privacy protection laws, this cookie policy page must be current and genuinely transparent about how the Website uses cookies and other tracking technologies when consumers visit there.

31. What is personally identifiable information (PII), and how do companies use it?

In democratic societies, it is common for citizens to feel that their PII is safeguarded from harm—whether the information exists on paper or online. To ensure that this is the case, jurisdictions adhering to this principle generally have a Privacy Commissioner Office that sets privacy protection policies and compliance guidelines. It also investigates complaints when provisions in existing Privacy Protection laws are perceived to have been broken.

To this critical end, if businesses are collecting PII from consumers to customize a better business experience for them, they need to be transparent about what the business purpose for collecting the PII is and how it will be safeguarded. An example of a company's being possibly non-compliant might occur when an online user files a complaint with the Privacy Commissioner Office, alleging that a particular social media site, say, said that they collect PII from users to give them a more positive online experience—but then share it with a third party for a totally different and undisclosed purpose.

By definition, Personal Information (PI), or PII, is consistently defined in privacy protection laws as information about an identifiable individual, where it reasonably can be assumed that a person can be identified through the use of that information alone (such as your Social Security Number), or in combination with other available PI (like your Driver's Licence Number and birth date).

In the past several years, what has become particularly threatening to citizens' privacy rights is the exponential growth in ransomware exploits on industry, government, and school district networks. These ill-motivated exploits inevitably place our PII in harm's way of some very bad actors, despite IT safeguards being in place. Particularly disturbing is when these ransomware gangs put troves of stolen PII on the Dark Web for other like-minded bad actors to use as they see fit for their own financial gain.

To illustrate the complexity of catching and bringing to justice these gangs inhabiting the bowels of the Dark Web, on April 5, 2023, an intriguing media piece in *The Guardian* described a sting led by the FBI, the Dutch police, and law enforcement agencies in eighteen countries that took down *Genesis Market*. As innocent as it sounds, *Genesis Market* was not a privacy-protecting entity but a criminal online marketplace on the Dark Web that sold millions of stolen identities for as little as $0.70 and as much as hundreds of US dollars—depending on the type and quantity of "quality" PII available. According to the authorities orchestrating this multi-jurisdictional privacy-protection sting, there were at least 80 million sets of personal credentials for sale in this marketplace, representing about 2 million unique online users. In fact, the PII stolen from various hack attacks on networks controlled by banks, *Facebook*, *Amazon*, *PayPal*, and *Netflix* were on sale here, along with the digital fingerprints from numerous victims' devices, enabling the bad guys to bypass online security checks by pretending to be the victims (i.e., identity theft).

Nevertheless, there is a "good news" ending to this real-life story of cyber fraud and other nefarious activities meant to "pad" the bad actors' wallets. The UK's National Crime Agency (NCA), a key player in this sting operation, said that they immediately arrested nineteen suspected bad actors in their jurisdiction known to frequent this marketplace. On a global scale, there were about 120 other suspected bad actors arrested after over 200 searches were completed by law enforcement across numerous jurisdictions. This real-life modern-day story underscores the importance of encouraging businesses, Privacy Commission Offices, and law enforcement to work hand-in-hand to help safeguard networks and to respond quickly when the PII of consumers and employees is at known Real Risk of Significant Harm because of hack attacks.

Besides the seriousness of present-day ransomware exploits, there is a growing phenomenon of concern less well known called "doxing," defined as the practice of publishing someone's PII online without their consent. Given the importance of the notion of Free Speech in democratic societies globally, the online environment has provided a convenient venue for doxing to be used increasingly as an intimidation tactic against targeted online users, setting the stage for acts like online vigilantism and land-based violence.

32. Can your smartphone track where you go, and who might be using this information?

Yes, your smartphone can track where you go in several ways, including through the apps you install and use. Geo-location tracking is done using cell towers and wireless networks. Whether you have an iPhone or Android device, your location is determined by your carrier's network infrastructure—which is non-intrusive to you as a user. As soon as you turn on your smartphone, it automatically connects to this infrastructure.

How can someone track you? By determining which cell towers you are closest to, someone trying to track your location can use a method called triangulation. So even if you're not making any calls or sending any texts or email messages, your phone will still routinely "check in" with the cell towers. In less urban areas, GPS can be also used by someone to locate you, and in more crowded areas like big cities, someone can track you using wi-fi, because your phone routinely scans for locations of access points. In fact, it is for this reason that IT security experts recommend that you either turn off your wi-fi when you want to be "location-anonymous" or use a virtual private network (VPN) to hide your IP address.

In short, IT security experts caution smartphone users that like all data connected online, our mobile phone location information can be used by the good guys for legitimate reasons—like authorities trying to locate us during an emergency, or by the bad guys for nefarious reasons.

How can you *disable* the location tracker on your smartphone? On an Android phone, the quickest way to do this is to go to the "Quick Settings" panel above your notifications heading, or open the "Settings" menu and find the "location settings" under the "Security" and "Privacy" headings. Not only can you disable your location data altogether using the latter method (and risk losing access to *Google Maps*), but you can also see which apps have recently made requests about your location. If you have an iPhone, the quickest way to disable your location tracker is to ask Siri to disable it, but you can also open the "Settings" app, scroll down to find the "Privacy" heading, and then toggle on or off the "Location Services."

On another cautionary note, some companies may ask you to download and deploy a location tracking app to enhance your buying experience. However, this data can be misused by the company and you may not even be aware of this fact. A summer 2022 case making media headlines for all the wrong reasons was the *Toronto-based Restaurant Brands International Inc.*, which owns the hugely popular Tim Horton's coffee and donut franchise in Canada. An investigation led by the federal Privacy Commissioner in response to a multiple class-action lawsuit found that the company violated Canadian Privacy Protection laws from April 2019 through September 2020 by collecting too much tracking data on consumers.

How? The company and its third-party partner tracked consumers' locations on their mobile phones even though users were told that the app would only be deployed in-store to alert users when their order was ready. Evidence showed that the app actually tracked millions of consumers' locations hundreds of times a day—even when the app was not open on their phones. While the company was told that they would have to change their privacy practices to be compliant with the law and delete any geo-location data collected during this period, it faced no fines or financial penalties for the noncompliance. As compensation to eligible app users whose privacy was invaded, they were able to claim a free hot beverage and a baked good when the investigation was completed.

Finally, over the past year, new legislation is starting to appear in some jurisdictions obligating employers to disclose how they conduct electronic surveillance of their employees—a workplace concern that came to light during Covid-19 lockdowns. For example, as of October 2022, all provincially regulated employers of Ontario, Canada, with twenty-five or more workers are required to have a written policy on how they monitor their employees—and how they might be using this information gathered from workplace surveillance. Importantly, the surveillance policy not only has to be shared with current and new employees, but any time an employer introduces new software or tools to track a worker without their knowledge, that information has to be shared with the employees. A movement is on, as well, to allow Canada's Office of the Privacy Commissioner to access employers' workplace surveillance policies to ensure that they are compliant with existing federal privacy protection laws.

33. Should you be concerned about your privacy or security when you interact with friends in social media sites?

For years, mental health experts have warned that over-using technology in any of its forms can lead to online addiction. Now add social media to the health risk category, particularly as it relates to users' privacy and security.

The controversy around social media risks surfaced loud and clear in October 2021 when *Facebook* whistleblower Frances Haugen told US Congress that when researchers and lawmakers asked how this US-based social media platform affects the privacy, health, and safety of teens actively engaged on it, the company was never forthcoming about the known dangers uncovered by their own research. Instead, it chose to mislead and misdirect any accountability for the harms to users. Haugen's testimony set off a very heated debate and a renewed interest by lawmakers in the United States, Canada, and elsewhere about how to safeguard teens when they go on social media sites to connect with friends. Let's look more closely at what is driving lawmakers' concerns from a privacy and security perspective—and what they are planning to do about it.

First, there is the security risk to users. Lawmakers argue that there are too many known cases of harm, such as that of Canadian teen Amanda Todd, who was cyber-stalked, cyber harassed, and cyber extorted for two years by an adult Dutch man. He would engage in social media platforms to lure her and other teen victims to perform online sexual acts for his own pleasure. Sadly, Amanda and others in similar circumstances have committed suicide to end their intense psychological pain and humiliation. Given the awful plight of these young victims, lawmakers maintain that we as a civilized society have agreed to not let a fifteen-year-old go to a land-based bar or a strip club, so why not have the same security protections in place when young people go online? Also, parents should be able to go to bed at night knowing that their children or teens are not looking at hard-core pornography or being lured by some nefarious adult hanging out in social media.

To address these security concerns, lawmakers seem intent on passing new pieces of legislation that have "more teeth." For example, in late April 2023, four US senators introduced the Protecting Kids on Social Media Act. If passed, it will not only require social media companies to verify users' ages—barring children younger than age thirteen from gaining access, but obtaining parental consent for access in the 13–17 age range. Laurie Schlegal, the Louisiana state representative spearheading this law's passage, said she was inspired to act after hearing a podcast hosted by broadcaster Howard Stern in which singer Billie Eilish declared that watching online porn as a child destroyed her brain. She said that the digital world needs the same kind of "adult zones" as those existing in the land-based world, where consumers are asked to show a government ID to buy alcohol, gamble online, or have alcohol delivered to their homes.

Nonetheless, civil liberties advocates in the United States have counter-argued that some of these proposed restrictions could inadvertently create age-verification barriers for netizens wanting to freely access information or communicate with friends online, including teens. If passed, these rules would, in fact, radically alter the Freedom of Information aspects of the internet by causing the online world to become a patchwork of seemingly "walled-off fiefdoms." It could also potentially cause popular social media or video platforms like *Facebook*, *X*, or *TikTok* to narrow their offerings to avoid charges of legal non-compliance. These alterations in virtual space, maintain these civil liberties advocates, would result in unreasonable prohibitions to online information or social media access for minors and adults, alike.

In Canada and in the European Union (EU), there is an equally active movement by lawmakers to push for stronger privacy safeguards for teens when they go on social media or other high-tech company platforms. The lawmakers in Canada, for example, want to pass new stricter laws so that young users' PII is not unnecessarily collected, distributed, or abused by social media or other high-tech companies just to make huge profits through targeted advertising (i.e., ads based on information shared by users to be able to obtain platform access). To this end, in June 2022, the Canadian Innovation Minister tabled a bill (called C-27) to enact the Consumer Privacy Protection Act. If passed, it would introduce some of the biggest fines in the world for high-tech companies found to be non-compliant with privacy protection legislation. In fact, fines could run as high as $25 million, or 5 percent of a company's global revenue, for *each* confirmed privacy law infringement. This Act would also increase the powers of Canada's Office of the Privacy Commissioner to investigate complaints made by teens or their parents and include convenient mechanisms for teens to request the deletion of their personal data without having to go to court or obtain a legal representative.

So, are there any recent legal precedents that would suggest that online users' privacy protection complaints against "big tech" companies actually result in real-world remedies in favor of the complainant? Yes, there is an interesting Canadian court case that was completed in September 2023, where the complainant, an adult male, wanted the Privacy Commissioner to take on US-based *Google* for infringement of Canada's existing privacy protection law—the Personal Information Protection and Electronic Documents Act, or PIPEDA. The man (whose identity is protected by law) argued that outdated and inaccurate information about him appearing in newspaper articles years ago was fed into *Google* searches by the company's algorithm. The result, he argued, was that he suffered tremendous mental, physical and privacy harms—including physical assault, employment discrimination, social stigma, and unrelenting fear. After filing his complaint with the Office of Privacy Commissioner, he asked the courts to order *Google* to remove the harmful content and have his name made unsearchable (legally known as "the right to be forgotten").

Google's defense team argued that the company merely acted as an intermediary between publishers and their audience, much like libraries do, and that they should be exempted from PIPEDA regulations. *Google* is just organizing the world's information to make it universally accessible to online users, argued the defense team in court, because netizens have "a right to know." In the end, in a 2-1 ruling, Canada's Federal Court of Appeal affirmed that *Google*, responsible for about 75 percent of online searches in Canada, is *not* covered by any exemption to PIPEDA. The justices ruled, in fact, that in this jurisdiction, there needs to be a case-by-case *balancing act* between the "public's right to know" and the "privacy of online citizens." In short, the complainant won his case, and *Google* had to make his name unsearchable.

34. What are targeted ads?

Targeted, or personalized ads, can be sent to you in one of two common ways. The first is by advertisers who have paid their branding fee to a high-tech platform like *Facebook* or *Instagram*. If you've ever clicked "accept all" to a tracking cookie notice on a given website, then you've actually consented to receiving targeted ads! The second way that you can receive targeted ads is by being active on a website or online forum promoting a particular topic of interest—and where nefarious peddlers of harmful products are likely to reside. In recent years, online forums offering advice on suicide methods as well or "pro-ana" and "thin-spiration" websites encouraging anorexia and other eating disorders have become quite popular among teens struggling with mental health issues.

In an effort to curb mental and physical harms to minors, various jurisdictions globally have passed or are considering passing tougher laws to counter the so-called "surveillance capitalism" and hyper-personalized ads that have become an inescapable part of users' seemingly one-sided social contract with Big-Tech companies. The motivation behind these laws is that high-tech companies need to "balance" users' safeguards with their commitment to give online users open access to information or social interaction.

Some jurisdictions are viewed as more progressive and more ahead of the curve than others. For example, in 2018, the EU passed progressive, landmark privacy legislation known as the General Data Protection Regulation (GDPR). This law created very strong privacy and security obligations for high-tech companies around the collection, retention, and management of users' personal data—including ruling that these companies cannot force online users to accept personalized ads without their explicit consent.

In terms of case relevance regarding personalized ad violations of the General Data Protection Regulation, in 2023, EU regulators found that *Meta* (who owns *Facebook* and *Instagram*) had actually been subverting the regulation's requirement for personalized ads. Therefore, they hit *Meta* with over $560 million worth of privacy fines! This recent EU ruling shows that not only is it possible to stand up to Big-Tech companies' predatory business practices, but it also reinforces the message that this significant penalty should act as a catalyst for privacy advocates and lawmakers in multiple jurisdictions to pass long overdue privacy reforms to better protect teens and minors from privacy and security harms because of these targeted ads.

But are the high-tech companies heeding this message? Are they, in fact, providing better protections by changing their business practices or algorithms to better safeguard young people when they go online? Apparently there is some progress on this front. *Google,* for example, has recently affirmed that its automated systems are now designed to stop online users from being exposed unexpectedly to harmful or shocking platform content, including these targeted ads. A spokesperson for the company there said that if users come to *Google* to search for information about "self-harm," they now see features promoting prevention hotlines that can provide users with critical help and support. The platform also apparently now blocks auto-complete predictions for those searches in an effort to *balance* safety and privacy safeguards for online users with the platform's commitment to give users open access to information.

In addition, the *Meta* spokesperson said that this high-tech company has revised its policies to strike a *balance* between stopping users from seeing sensitive or upsetting content and giving them online space to talk about their experiences. This change in policy apparently occurred after mental health experts advised *Meta* that removing content about suicide and eating disorders could make troubled users to feel even more isolated. The spokesperson also said that the platform tries to remove harmful content/ads encouraging suicide, self-harm, or eating disorders, especially content offering suicide methods or instructions for drastic weight loss.

What happens to known nefarious peddlers of poisons in websites and online forums? Do they get away with pushing their harmful targeted ads or content, or are they sanctioned through criminal charges? A recent 2023 case of a Canadian peddler selling a potentially lethal product over the internet has begun to shed some light on these intriguing questions.

The substance peddled was sodium nitrate, a salt derivative used in very small quantities to cure meat. However, apparently ingesting just one spoon of this substance can result in someone's death. The perpetrator charged is a 57-year-old man named Kenneth Law. A former engineer and hotel chef in Toronto, Law was arrested and criminally charged under the Canadian Criminal Code with counseling suicide in the deaths of at least two Canadians. He is also suspected of sending lethal shipments of sodium nitrate to at least seven other deceased victims globally, including a seventeen-year-old boy in the United States and four British citizens in their twenties and thirties.

In fact, a recent British coroner's report submitted to the prosecution suggests that one of the deceased believed to have purchased the sodium nitrate was a 23-year-old British woman who apparently had frequented online communities of people openly discussing suicide. While the case against Law has yet to be heard and any sanctions levied, there appear to be few, if any, protections at this point afforded to vulnerable online users exposed to these targeted ads or who, consequently, make the lethal substance purchases peddled there.

35. What purpose do Terms of Service (ToS) associated with social networking sites serve?

Terms of Service (ToS) associated with social networking or other online platforms are generally meant to delineate behaviors deemed to be unacceptable if a user wants to continue engaging in that virtual space. Besides complying with existing legislative provisions in various jurisdictions, the ToS of social media platforms often also contain their own customized stipulations regarding unwanted activities and the consequences for users if these activities are detected.

As a case in point, the Statement of Rights and Responsibilities section of *Facebook*'s ToS deems unacceptable activities to include bullying, intimidating, or harassing any other user; posting content that is hate speech, is threatening, or is pornographic; posting content to incite violence; or posting content that contains nudity or graphic violence and exceeds the community standards. In short, this ToS section emphasizes that users cannot use the social media platform to do anything unlawful, misleading, malicious, or discriminatory.

If users are found to be violating *Facebook*'s ToS, what happens next? The Protecting Other People's Rights section underscores the point that the platform respects other people's rights, and all users are expected to do the same. To this end, users will not post content or take any action on the platform that infringes or violates someone else's rights or otherwise violates the law. If complaints are received that certain users are being noncompliant, the platform *can remove any content or information the users post if the adjudicators believe it violates this section of the ToS or the platform's broader policies.*

In support of Free Speech, *Facebook's* Community Standards section of the ToS states that while the platform does not tolerate bullying or harassment, it encourages users to speak freely on matters or people of public interest. However, the platform will take swift action regarding all reports of abusive behavior directed at individual users. For example, *repeatedly* targeting another user with unwanted friend requests or messages is considered by the platform to be an unacceptable form of harassment. The platform also does not permit hate speech or other users' or groups' attacking individuals based on their race, ethnicity, national origin, religion, sex, gender, sexual orientation, disability, or medical condition. The platform also strictly prohibits the sharing of pornographic content or content that is sexually explicit and involves a minor. Finally, while the platform places limits on content displaying nudity—it does permit some degree of nudity in content of personal importance, such as a woman's posting breastfeeding photos of her and her baby.

Generally speaking, "grey zones" regarding misinterpretation of social media ToS guidelines have been identified by experts. Here are four of the most frequent: (1) Because the ToS often contain a clause related to jurisdiction, significant conflict of law issues have arisen, leading to a problem in enforcement of the provision in certain jurisdictions; (2) the ToS may not be binding on minors, as they may not fully understand what is meant by the stipulated content; (3) when the ToS are deemed to be violated, users should report the abuse immediately (by using the "report abuse" button), prompting the platform to not only respond immediately but apply appropriate sanctions, if necessary; and (4) the ToS may include clauses denying liability for "inappropriate" content or activities by users in jurisdictions where such clauses are deemed to be invalid or unenforceable.

Generally speaking, how many reports of abuse have the social media and search engine platforms received from North American government regulators in recent years, and what is the predominant nature of these complaints? Interestingly, both *Google* and *Meta* publish public reports on how often different levels of government in various jurisdictions request removal of certain posts deemed to be inappropriate or offensive. *Google's* reporting shows that since 2011, for example, it has received 1,347 requests from Canadian government entities at all levels—federal, provincial, and municipal. The most recent data show that between January and June, 2022, *Google* (which also owns *YouTube*) removed seventy-three posts—mostly because of defamation, privacy and security concerns, inappropriate adult content, bullying, or harassment. For this same period, *Meta*'s data show that it restricted access to content following 2,859 requests from the Canadian government for a broad range of reasons.

Do the social media companies respond quickly to these government requests to remove alleged harmful content? Answer: Apparently only partially so. *Facebook, Instagram, X, TikTok,* and *LinkedIn* all complied quickly with certain Canadian government requests—particularly if the posts infringed copyright laws or the platform's policies. However, social media platforms often retained posts that the government alleged were offensive, maintaining that the posts should be allowed because of the platform's support of Free Speech.

36. What is sexting? Is it illegal to send sexts?

"Sexting" occurs when online users—often teens or pre-teens—write sexually explicit messages to other users, or take sexually explicit photos of themselves (or others in their peer group) and then transmit those photos and/or messages to their peers or love interests. In short, sexting refers to sexually explicit content communicated online via text messages or through online forums, including social media. The practice of sending sexually suggestive images is not limited to the younger online population; rather, adults also engage in this type of behavior as part of the dating or partnership cycle.

Mental health experts generally maintain that sexting is not illegal in most democratic jurisdictions but is, in fact, considered to be a normal part of young adults' expressing their sexuality. The key is that in most jurisdictions, legality is viewed as occurring when parties engaging in sexting activities do so with *consent*. Accepting this condition, experts generally distinguish between primary and secondary sexting. "Primary sexting" is when individuals intentionally take sexually explicit pictures of themselves and then share those with trusted peers online. "Secondary sexting" is when another party forwards or further shares a sexually explicit picture sent to him/her by the individual taking the picture—without that individual's consent. So, from a legal perspective, primary sexting is generally seen as consensual—unless it is the result of coercion by another person—in which case it is likely to be considered as illegal. Sexting may, in fact, be part of a cyberharassment, cyber extortion, or cyberstalking campaign by another online user—in which case criminal sanctions could apply because consent was not given but was coerced.

If asked, would the majority of teens view sexting as "healthy"? In an interesting 2014 study led by Professor Stefaan Walrave, about 500 students aged 15–18 in two Belgian high schools were asked whether they partook in sexting—and how they felt about doing so. About 26 percent of the teens surveyed had engaged in sexting in the two months preceding the study. Most had done so only once or a few times. How did they feel about doing so? The average score of respondents reflected a slightly negative attitude toward this activity—with perceived social pressure to do so by peers as their main motivating factor. Females also said that often they were pressured by their existing romantic partners or by their potential romantic partners to send sexts as part of the dating ritual. Professor Walrave suggested that to reduce sexting among adolescents, preventative initiatives should transparently disclose that many teens hold the view that sexting is not pleasant, particularly if it is coercive in nature rather than consensual.

37. What can you do if you're receiving unwanted sexts?

Sexting is when someone writes sexually explicit messages or takes sexually explicit photos of themselves or others in their peer group and then transmits those to another online user or set of online users. From a legal perspective, sexting can either be consensual and legal or coerced and illegal.

So, what are your options if you're receiving *unwanted* sexts from someone? Basically, you have three options: (1) Submit a complaint to the source—say *Facebook*—through the "report abuse" button; (2) submit a complaint to a school counselor or other designated school health professional, who will be assigned to see you through this problem and provide you with the necessary safety interventions; and/or (3) submit a complaint to the police and be truthful about what you know about the unwanted sexting messages or coerced demands if they are brought in to resolve your case or lay criminal charges against the perpetrator.

Professionals or authorities assigned to your case will likely ask you questions pertaining to the incident, like: Do you know who was involved in the production and distribution of the sexting message, and how many people received it? What kind of sexting message was sent to you (e.g., a text message, a partially nude photo, a fully nude photo, a depiction of sexual intercourse, or screenshots of sexual activities)? What was the context of the sexting message (e.g., a form of flirtation, part of an existing or previous intimate relationship, or an attempt to extort money or bully you)? Was the unwanted message forwarded to your friends or posted on a specific website or platform?

After assessing your situation, the school counselor or police will work with you to create a strategy for quickly and safely dealing with the immediate harms, to stop the spread of the sexting message to others, and to collect and keep evidence if the courts become involved and criminal charges are indeed filed.

Finally, it is important to note that a number of US states have special sexting legislation in place. As of March 2023, for example, these states have it: Arizona, Arkansas, Connecticut, Colorado, Florida, Georgia, Hawaii, Indiana, Illinois, Kansas, Louisiana, Nebraska, Nevada, New Jersey, New Mexico, New York, North Dakota, South Dakota, Oklahoma, Pennsylvania, Rhode Island, Tennessee, Texas, Utah, Vermont, and West Virginia. Where special sexting laws are not in place, criminal cases will typically be heard under existing laws dealing with child pornography. Importantly, the criminal offense level of sexting varies from state to state, with the more lenient jurisdictions treating the first instance of sexting by a minor as a noncriminal offense but subjecting a reoffending minor to criminal prosecution.

38. What should you do if you receive obscene messages from someone online?

If you live in North America and you are receiving offensive, obscene messages from someone online, what are your options? David Butt, a trial and appellate lawyer in Toronto, Canada, and a graduate of Harvard Law School, shares this legal perspective. In democratic societies, "obscenity" is a legal term applying to anything deemed to be offensive to society's morals because of its indecency or lewdness. In North America, for example, "obscenity" and "obscene content" have often been equated with pornography and child pornography. However, obscenity law is constantly evolving, and what was considered to be shocking content fifty years, twenty years, or a decade ago may not be perceived as shocking by most citizens today. Given this reality, the courts must constantly revisit obscenity laws to ensure that they keep pace with modern standards. That is why most contemporary obscenity laws in North America use a standard known as "the community standard of tolerance."

In applying this standard, judges look to the prevailing values of a community—which may be delineated by expert witnesses called into court. In light of this testimony, judges will assess what sort of materials or messages are so bad so as to not only be "distasteful" but "intolerable" by the community. In short, criminalizing only "intolerable" material or messages has the effect of preserving as much as possible broad freedoms of expression enjoyed by citizens on land and online.

Those feeling victimized by obscene and/or offensive content online have a variety of legal options—which have increased in recent years as lawmakers come to understand how and why online victimization is a pressing social problem. Basically, the options available to victims are categorized into two: (1) criminal remedies and (2) civil remedies. If the online content is so offensive that it not only violates an applicable criminal law in that jurisdiction but that it seems to exceed the community standard of tolerance, the victim can report the incident to police. The police will then take over the investigation, and if there is enough compelling evidence, the alleged perpetrator will be charged by the prosecutor with various counts under the Criminal Code. The case would then be put before the courts. If there is a conviction and the perpetrator is found "guilty" on some or all of the charges, the judge can put the offender in jail and/ or order appropriate compensation for the victim.

Second, a person suffering from victimization can also sue the perpetrator civilly. This procedure requires hiring a lawyer to carry forward the lawsuit. In civil proceedings, the perpetrator will not be convicted of a criminal offense and will not go to jail. Instead, he or she will be ordered by the court to pay money, or damages, to the victim to compensate for the harm suffered and to make the victim "whole." The court can also order the perpetrator to cease and desist victimizing the target. Notably, if the perpetrator fails to be compliant, he or she can eventually be placed behind bars.

39. What are piracy websites and who uses them?

Piracy websites offer illegal downloads or streaming of copyrighted content. Many of these websites are housed in the Dark Web, where you would need to not only understand but use BitTorrent technology to access the goods available. So if you're interested in viewing blockbuster movies like *Top Gun: Maverick*, superhero epics like *Thor: Love and Thunder*, or romantic comedies like *The Lost City*, you can find them on these piracy websites—for free. If you're wondering how much these piracy websites impact global economies, professionals estimate that the costs to the US economy, alone, likely range from $29 billion to $71 billion.

In fact, many of these present-day piracy websites now operate as streamers themselves—packaged with monthly subscription rates for a wide range of high-demand, illegal content. They also appear to be collecting tons of online advertising revenue—just like legal entities like *Facebook* or *X*. In fact, Bloomberg estimates that the piracy websites' advertising revenues could be as high as $1+ billion a year.

Who uses these piracy websites and how often? As a case in point, according to the Motion Picture Association (MPA) of Canada, there were an estimated 3.8 billion visits to these illegal websites by Canadians in 2020. Furthermore, the MPA says that about 12 percent of Canadian households actually had subscriptions to TV piracy services in 2020, an increase from 9 percent in 2019—which seems to a trend rather than an exception.

In what jurisdictions is illegal downloading of copyrighted works occurring most frequently, you may ask? Michael Bachmann, a Criminology professor at Texas Christian University, says that statistics show it tends to occur most often in these countries: Brazil, France, the United States, Canada, and Britain. Consequently, he calls illegal downloading "a First World phenomenon," despite existing laws passed to combat piracy, such as the Digital Millennium Copyright Act (DMCA) passed in the United States.

What's more, Professor Bachmann adds, accurately quantifying such illegal online activities on a global scale is an extremely difficult undertaking, resulting in a woeful lack of useful information for crime prevention. He says that the reason that streaming, or "torrenting," of large movie files is so prominent in developed economies is that being able to do so requires access to a high-speed broadband connection—most commonly found in Western countries. What's more, the music and movies generally protected under copyright protection laws like the DMCA are produced primarily in English, with Western consumers not only in mind for marketing but for demand.

So what's being done to help combat illegal downloading in these jurisdictions? Professor Bachmann says that while there are a number of options, consumer education about this criminal behavior is critical. For example, colleges and universities often post "illegal file-sharing policies" on their websites for students to understand that this behavior will not be tolerated. However, he adds, it's not just the posting of these policies that is effective but the active monitoring and sometimes even throttling or blocking of typical torrent ports on campus. By exercising proactive due diligence, these colleges and universities can arguably be in a more favorable position in cases of future litigation by the creative holders or legitimate distributors of the copyrighted material.

Law enforcement, as well, have become actively engaged in the fight against piracy websites, coordinating with one another across jurisdictions and borders.

For example, with codenames like "Operation Krypton" and "Operation 404," law enforcement in multiple jurisdictions have been able to seize 24,000 illicit devices in Madrid and shut down 226 piracy websites and 461 piracy apps in Brazil. Also, in March, 2023, three popular illegal services operating in three provinces in Canada (i.e., the Ontario-based Northern IPTV, the Quebec-based IPTVOnline24, and the Alberta-based GloryV) were not only shut down by the authorities but their domains were redirected to the MPA's (Motion Pictures Association's) "Watch Legally" website.

Finally, like colleges and universities, copyright protection advocates like the MPA are trying to educate consumers. Their message is loud and clear: That the real-world criminals operating piracy websites are the same ones engaging in other illegal activities on the Dark Web—including gambling, money laundering, tax evasion, drug sales, grand theft auto, human trafficking, and prostitution. What's more, emphasize these advocates, rampant piracy likely means that creative film companies may not be able to finance their next movie—which means that more people in the creative industry will lose their jobs. In fact, it's not just about the large studios being negatively impacted—it's about the potential downfall of the entire entertainment industry ecosystem.

40. Is it illegal to share your streaming service logins with friends or family?

Streaming is a technology used to deliver content to your computer or mobile devices over the internet without having to download it. So, you may wonder, if you are a legitimate streaming subscriber, is it illegal for you to share your streaming service logins with friends or family members? Answer: Yes, it is illegal to share your streaming service logins with friends or family *if it violates your service provider's Terms of Service (ToS).*

In other words, violating your provider's stated policy means that you are engaging in piracy—which is not only illegal in North American jurisdictions (and elsewhere) because it violates existing copyright laws—but that your mooching causes a major profit loss to the streaming service. Because your streaming service may allow you to do simultaneous streaming on multiple devices you own—you may falsely believe that you can share your service logins with any number of friends or family members. However, the best advice is this: Closely read your ToS to determine if there are any limits to "legal login sharing" in your provider's policy.

For example, *Amazon Prime* says on its website that its policy on "legally sharing accounts/logins" is governed by its Amazon Household feature—which is defined as legal sharing of up to ten people living under one household roof. *FuboTV*, in contrast, allows only two devices to stream at the same time, and if a user exceeds this legal limit, he or she will be prompted to pay an additional $5.99 subscription fee to add another. Like *Amazon Prime*, *Hulu* is okay with login sharing with others living within the same household, but login sharing is not allowed with individuals living outside the home. Finally, *PhiloTV* appears to have one of the more forgiving policies when it comes to account sharing, because a user is not required to enter a so-called "home account." Rather, up to three devices in different locations can legally stream at the same time, but if a user tries to add a fourth device in another location, the earliest stream will be shut down!

So who is reportedly the most guilty demographic exceeding these allowable limits and letting friends mooch without paying for the streaming service? According to recent statistics cited by the finance news site CNBC, 35 percent of millennials share their login passwords with others in violation of their provider's policy limits, 19 percent of Gen X subscribers do, and 13 percent of Baby Boomers do. Consequently, streaming service providers find themselves with significant business losses annually. *Hulu*, for example, argues that they lose around $1.5 billion a year due to illegal mooching.

Now, here is a final cautionary note: Subscribers breaching their contractual terms and allowing others to mooch can find themselves having to pay a damages claim from their streaming platform because of these significant profit losses. The streaming platform may also terminate or restrict a legitimate user's account when the violation occurs.

41. Is it illegal to download and share copyrighted files like songs or movies?

Downloading and then sharing copyrighted files like music or movies from online distribution sites offering these works to you for free is illegal in most democratic jurisdictions because of infringement of existing Copyright Protection laws. In the United States, for example, the copyright law protecting creators' rights related to the legal reproduction and performance of their works is the federal Digital Millennium Copyright Act (DCMA).

Regardless of jurisdiction, the overarching purpose of copyright laws is to *balance* creators' and users' rights by securing just rewards for the creators (known as royalties), while facilitating public access to these works. When this balance is achieved, not only is society enriched, but the creators are encouraged to produce more works. Users also gain by having legal access to these works—which they can then use to inspire their own original artistic and intellectual creations. Furthermore, these laws protect the creators and users by ensuring that the works attract the same rights and provide the same royalties *regardless of the technological means* used to legally distribute these works. Similar to off-line distributions, users who legally download or stream works maintain this intended balance.

Why? Because under most copyright laws, a work is "performed" as soon as it is made available for on-demand streaming—and at this point, a royalty fee is paid to the creator by the legal distributor. If the work is later *legally* streamed by a user—who pays a subscription fee to the distributer, no additional royalty is paid to the creator, because the stream is part of what is known as "a continuous act of performance" that began when the work was originally made available to the public.

Besides infringing the balancing purpose of copyright law protections, online users engaging in illegal downloading and file-sharing can also cause major security issues for their school's or their employer's network, as illustrated by the current barrage of costly ransomware attacks reported by schools and businesses. Also, violating copyright laws (like the DMCA) can result in serious civil and criminal lawsuit penalties for those found to be responsible for the infringement.

For example, in a civil lawsuit, the infringer could be liable to pay the copyright owner's actual damages plus any profits made from the infringement. Or the copyright owner could elect to accept a statutory damage recovery fee from the infringer of up to $150,000—if the court decides that the infringement was willful.

In a criminal lawsuit, if the infringer is convicted and found guilty of violating the DMCA, the sanctions applied in the United States will be based on the severity of the infringement and the number of times the perpetrator has breached the Act. For example, the first time an infringer illegally downloads and then distributes "during any 180-day period at least 10 illegal copies of copyrighted songs or movies with a retail value of more than $2,500," he or she can be imprisoned for up to five years and fined up to $250,000—or both. If the infringer has been previously convicted and found guilty of repeat copyright infringement, he or she could be sentenced to a maximum of ten years behind bars, a $250,000 fine—or both. Finally, if the infringer is found guilty of committing a misdemeanor (i.e., a less serious violation) of the DMCA—such as reproducing and distributing fewer than ten copies of the works, he or she could be sentenced to a maximum of one year behind bars and fined a maximum of $100,000.

42. How can you spot fake news and conspiracy theories, and is there a way to prevent individuals or websites from spreading misinformation?

Fake news is all around us, but how can we inoculate ourselves from buying-into it or spreading it? Let's begin by looking at some recent misinformation and fake news incidents and then discuss what the experts tell us is the psychology behind misinformation.

During the Covid-19 lockdowns, we were all tethered to our smartphones and computers to access the latest news on the spread of the virus and its spiraling death toll globally. Truth be told, we were bombarded with both preventative measures by public health authorities and lots of misinformation, fake news, and conspiracy theories about how the virus was created and who "let it loose" on society.

As the Covid-19 "fake news" cycle passed, there were other compelling news reports surfacing about how certain victims harmed by distributors of fake news sought remedies in court for the distress they experienced. One of these cases involved Houston lawyer Wes Ball, who successfully led a civil lawsuit against US talk radio personality Alex Jones for repeatedly spreading falsehoods on his show about the Sandy Hook mass shooting that killed twenty elementary school children and six adults. Jones, who said "it never happened," was found guilty of the charges brought against him by the parents of the deceased children and ordered to pay nearly $1 billion in damages by the court.

Add to this false information mix the civil lawsuit that erupted when lawyers for former President Trump accused Dominion Voting Systems of playing a key role in stealing the 2020 presidential election from him—a story repeated daily by hosts at Fox News. These accusations not only prompted death threats against Dominion's employees and local election officials but fueled a defamation case by Dominion against Fox News for "knowingly spreading lies." In the end, in

2023, Fox Corporation and Fox News settled the defamation lawsuit by agreeing to pay Dominion Voting Systems $785.5 million, averting a trial at the eleventh hour but putting one of the world's top media companies in the legal crosshairs over its coverage of false vote-rigging claims.

Besides fake news, 2023 brought in some interesting fake news ads generated by Artificial Intelligence (AI) capabilities. For example, in a somewhat amusing incident, *TikTok* showed a video ad of comedian Joe Rogan and his guest endorsing a so-called libido-boosting coffee brand for men. Some viewers were amused by the video, while others were shocked—including Rogan's guest, who argued that the video ad was a fake. This fake ad is actually indicative of a growing number of fake videos shown on social media—and in response, some social media platforms have begun to take action. For example, *TikTok* has amended its policies to prohibit digital forgeries that mislead users by distorting the truth of events and causing significant harm to the video's featured subject, other persons, or society. *Meta* and *Twitch* have also banned "deep fake" and manipulative videos meant to deceive users.

So how can online users spot misinformation, false news, or deep fakes to safeguard themselves from intentional manipulation? For starters, users need to understand the psychological forces driving misinformation. According to psychologists, conspiracy theories and fake news flourish during events shaking our sense of security and altering our lives considerably. Humans engage in what they call "collective sense-making." Simply put, humans tend to work with others and to "think out loud" to better understand and give meaning to what is happening to us and around us. As part of this process, suppositions made by some individuals can snowball into conspiracy theories or "pseudoscience." In fact, affirm psychologists, conspiracy theories not believed in times of peace and serenity often flourish in non-normative times—such as during the Covid-19 pandemic, because we tend to attribute "large events" to "large causes."

During these periods of high anxiety, humans not only tend to gravitate toward like-minded people and the information they are "buying-into," but routinely engage in social media sites or listen to news networks (like Fox News or CNN) amplifying our preferred views. We essentially become "information hobbits," comfortable and satisfied with our believed "truths." We may even act out online with some degree of verbal hostility toward differing points of view and the people who espouse them. Or, we may become so radicalized that we verbally and physically exhibit hostility toward opposing factions—at which point psychologists might label us as "information hooligans."

So how does the opposing faction influence us to move over to their side? Again, experts say that conspiracy theories, in particular, erupt to erode our faith in public institutions and our trust in experts' data-driven advice. In fact, the opposing faction hopes that the more often we hear a false statement, the more believable it will sound to us. And the more people believe that something is true, the more likely they will share it with others. In fact, it is interesting to note that in 2018, MIT researchers analyzed *Twitter* data and estimated that it actually takes the truth about six times longer than a lie to reach around 1,500 online users! What's more, misinformation that inspires negative emotions in us—particularly disgust and fear—travels the fastest in social media!

So how can we verify that news is "real" and not fake? Answer: through *fact-checking*. In recent years, independent fact-checking websites and services have appeared to help combat fake news and fake news hooligans. But while fact-checking can help those who maintain an open mind in their search for truth and myth-busting, research also suggests that, not surprisingly, fake news hooligans tend to avoid fact-checking protocols.

Sander van der Linden, a world-leading expert on misinformation at the University of Cambridge, says that we can protect ourselves from misinformation with a promising concept he calls "psychological inoculation." His theory is that a sort of pre-bunking "vaccine" involving fact-checking *and* critical thinking can prime our brains to recognize and reject fake news. By becoming immune to misinformation's persuasive ploys, we are not only less vulnerable to accept it but less likely to spread it—because as informed humans, we feel less gullible and less vulnerable. Therefore, we are better able to turn off misinformation and fake news. This expert cites a much earlier piece of research suggesting that American soldiers could be protected from brainwashing by the enemy if they were taught psychological inoculation strategies to deflect it.

To help online users become better inoculated, he and colleagues have created a series of *YouTube* videos to enhance critical thinking immunity and free online games (called "Bad News" and "Bad News Junior") to help users better understand and spot a number of tricks often used to bait us—including fake experts, scary emotional language, and scapegoating others. After playing these games, he posits that online users have boosted their relative immunity against misinformation by at least 25 percent.

Addressing Technology Over-Use

43. What does "being mindful about technology use" really mean?

"Mindful technology use" means being intentional about how we use technology—typically our smartphones and our computers—and being acutely aware of how its over-use can negatively affect our mental health, our physical health, and our overall well-being. Being "mindful" also means being able to step back from constant mental and visual stimulation to play online games, to text others on our smartphones, or to binge-watch our favorite tv shows on our computers. Mental health experts maintain that we need to put our devices away for a while and on a regular basis to learn to be present "in the moment." By building a mindful use of technology paradigm into our life routines, posit these experts, we can enjoy healthier long-term relationships not only with technology (to continue enjoying what it enables us to do) but with land-based friends and family members.

How can you become more mindful about technology use? Here are some guidelines experts suggest: (1) Use only one device or app at a time; (2) limit your screen time to two hours or less daily, if possible; (3) park your smartphone in another room other than in your bedroom before retiring for the night so as not to be tempted to read email or text others when you should be sleeping; (4) disconnect from all of your blue screens at least one hour before bedtime; and (5) analyze your technology use weekly—and following this monitoring, if you believe that you are over-using technology and can't make a change in your routine on your own (no matter how many times you've tried), consider seeing a mental health professional for possible addiction assessment and useful assistance in regaining your life balance.

In short, warn mental health experts, happiness is not found on a blue screen but on land—the result of our interacting with real people and experiencing real life events that enhance our happiness and well-being. Happiness can't be derived from the number of *Facebook* "Likes" we've just received. In fact, our digitally produced sources of nearly everything—from information to possible love partners—can also become our leading source of falsehood and loneliness. A disturbing chart looking at the behavior of US high school teens shows that, as their internet use soared a decade ago, their in-person socializing dropped, their sleep worsened, and their happiness plummeted.

44. What exactly is a "digital detox," and what are the costs and benefits?

According to Narenda Kumar Pathak from the Indira Gandhi National Open University in India, a digital detox is deliberately switching off all smartphones, tablets, laptops, and computers for a certain length of time. Even though the science of how technology impacts human behavior is still in its infancy, digital detox as a concept, he notes, made its way into *The Oxford Dictionary* in 2013. The main purpose of a digital detox is to provide an online user with the opportunity to reduce his or her stress (particularly elevated levels of anxiety and depression) by focusing on social interactions and life experiences with others in the physical world rather than just relying on relationship-building in the virtual world.

While undergoing a digital detox means refraining from using online devices for a certain length of time, the designated detox period may also include refraining from using other more conventional items like tvs or work-related tools and programs. These restrictions apply to individuals regularly "unplugging" for the twenty-five hours of Shabbat—a practice that has existed in the observant Jewish community for centuries, where the use of electricity by community members is strictly forbidden on the weekly day of rest known as Shabbat. Interestingly, this law was derived from the saying, "You shall not kindle fire in any of your dwellings on Sabbath day."

In a broader sense, digital detox for the mainstream centers on the prevention of or remediation from various harms produced by excessive digital media usage. Reported harms include internet addiction as well as an unhealthy disconnect from family and friends in the land-based world. From a digital media perspective, digital detox is a phenomenon tapping into the promise of "authenticity," as it offers various ways to counter-experience "inauthenticity" in online interactions, particularly in social media. Research has consistently found that online interactions are perceived by online users to be faceless, factually inaccurate, and privacy-invading. Viewed in this light, digital detox is definitely a countermovement to inauthenticity.

How many online users have admitted to completing a digital detox? According to a pre-Covid lockdown survey conducted by marketing firm GWI in 2018, of over 4,000 respondents in Britain and the United States who took part in the self-report study, one in five (about 20 percent) said that they had completed a digital detox—with 70 percent confirming that they wanted to limit the time they spent online to help elevate their moods and become more engaged with friends and family in the land-based world.

Another recent study published in 2023 was conducted by an international team of researchers who examined data from 287,282 UK BioBank participants, including 13,000 individuals with serious cases of clinical depression. All of these participants were tracked for nine years. The researchers identified several healthy lifestyle factors associated with lower risk of depression, including (1) maintaining a healthy diet (by eating three servings of fruit and vegetables daily, eating fish at least twice a week, ingesting minimal amounts of processed foods and red meats, and consuming at least three servings of whole grains daily); (2) getting regular physical activity (by incorporating at least 150 minutes of moderate exercise a week), (3) routinely maintaining a healthy sleep pattern (by getting seven to nine hours of refueling sleep a night), (4) moderating alcohol intake, (5) not smoking, (6) decreasing sedentary behavior (by sitting less than four hours daily), and (7) maintaining frequent land-based social connections. Notably, these same healthy lifestyle habits are also touted in well-recognized digital detox programs globally.

Given that completing a digital detox routinely has a positive impact on our well-being and life happiness, what are the costs? The primary cost cited is the type of digital detox protocol individuals choose to experience. At the low-cost end are schools or community-based courses offering digital detox regimens, as well as self-help books written by mental health experts for successfully developing healthier tech habits. Also at the low-cost end but intended for those experiencing internet addiction is voluntary attendance at an Internet and Tech Addicts Anonymous (ITAA) group set of meetings, a fellowship program (similar to Alcoholics Anonymous) offering a "12-step connection" protocol designed to bring hope, resources, and personal support to those confronting the personal harms of tech addiction. At the higher-cost end is attendance at a specially designed digital detox resort (found in numerous domestic and exotic locales) or at the California-based Camp Grounded for adults wanting to do a three-day weekend detox with likeminded others. Also at the more costly end in terms of time and money (but worth every minute and penny) are specially designed mental health programs like that offered at the US-based Center for Internet Addiction—which typically require participants to undergo a digital detox before beginning treatment for their online addiction.

45. What is the digital detox manifesto?

In 2020, the opening quote on the US-based Digital Detox Company's website posited that there is an underlying premise that emerging technologies should be created by companies mindfully and ethically so as to benefit its consumers, not harm them mentally, socially, or physically. Known as the "Digital Detox Manifesto," this premise was delineated like this:

> We believe that technologies should serve as tools to connect us … as we celebrate life, truly improving our unique existence, instead of distracting, disturbing, or disrupting us. And we believe that these technologies should be created mindfully and ethically, for the benefit of and not at the cost of consumers and users. In fact, the relationship that grows between the creator and consumer should be truly symbiotic and honest.

Basically, the digital detox manifesto calls for revisiting how we humans relate to the grid and to our digital devices. It imparts this clear message: Unless we curtail our current patterns of being digitally tethered for twenty-four hours, seven days a week, our stress levels will continue to climb, along with various forms of internet addiction. Half the solution, affirm the manifesto creators, is for netizens to mindfully develop new positive social norms and online etiquette. The other half of the solution is for technology companies to develop products that are created mindfully and ethically for the benefit of its users, not at the expense of their well-being or privacy. Maybe it is time, to conclude these manifesto creators, for both tech companies and online users to reflect on the authentic things in life that we nowadays seem to take for granted. In short, it is time for tech companies and online users to take a deep breath, pause, and remember that "we are all in this together."

But are technology companies following this manifesto to a tee?? Let's look at the evidence. In 2023 in the United States, a bipartisan posse of US lawmakers began to sharpen their sticks against *TikTok* and other social media companies like *Facebook* (witness the 2021 damning testimony on Capitol Hill by whistleblower

Frances Haugen) for not only ignoring this warning but surreptitiously putting online users' well-being and privacy in harm's way.

For *TikTok*, in particular, the US lawmakers argue that they want to ban it altogether in the United States—or at least force the platform's Chinese owners to sell their stakes in the company—out of fear it is actually a Chinese spying machine for the Chinese government. Its presence not only jeopardizes national security, the lawmakers posit, but presents a major well-being and privacy cost to US netizens.

As long as *TikTok* remains active in the US jurisdiction, which segment of users would appear to be at particular risk of personal harm? Answer: teens and young adults, who comprise a considerable portion of the *TikTok* follower cult. According to a recent release by Wallaroo Media, a significant 60 percent of the platform's faithful are under age thirty—and some are as young as ten. On average, young users reportedly open this app eight times a day, and 83 percent of them regularly post their own videos on the platform—showing them dancing or helping their dogs do tricks. For the more creative types using this platform to market their talent, the loss of the platform would be scary, for the "creatives" would quickly discover whether their presumed talent is driving their popularity—or if it's *TikTok*'s powerful algorithms driving it.

The loss of *TikTok* would also expose the truths on "the influencer" economy— promoted on this platform as well on other popular US-based platforms like *Facebook*, *YouTube*, and *Instagram*. To many, the conundrum remains as to exactly what credentials other than celebrity status or good looks most of these popular influencers really have. But in today's social-media-obsessed culture, minimal expertise appears to be satisfactory to many gullible online users.

At the end of the day, suggest advocates of the Digital Detox Manifesto, the loss of *TikTok* in the North American online scene would have many more benefits than just limiting China's potential viewing of users' personally identifiable data. But until and if that happens, other hugely popular social media platforms will likely pick up the slack—and the harmful cycle of mindless but addictive activity by users will unfortunately continue for the foreseeable future.

46. What is Internet and Tech Addicts Anonymous (ITAA)?

The Internet and Tech Addicts Anonymous (ITAA) group is a fellowship program for individuals, their partners, and their families who find themselves dealing with technology addiction. Like Alcoholics Anonymous (AA)—aimed at helping alcoholics, the ITAA is a fellowship program aimed at helping tech addicts. Founded in 2009, the ITAA's protocol is based on a twelve-step "connection" of the tech addict with others in the group. As well, a connection to a higher power is emphasized—to bring hope, resources, and personal support to members confronting the personal harms of tech addiction. Importantly, the ITAA is open to incorporating other program protocols—such as twelve-traditions or non-theistic ones. The benefit of this fellowship program is that it is a low-cost option for those wanting to heal from tech addiction, since no dues or fees are required to join. However, participants wanting to give contributions are welcome to do so at weekly meetings.

ITAA recognizes that along with a tech addiction is a tendency for tech addicts to conceal their heavy usage to the point that the actual amount of time spent interfacing with their computers, smartphones, or other tech gadgets is often minimized by them or denied altogether. So, the twelve-step protocol and principles emphasize things like the willingness of group members (1) To admit that their lives have become unmanageable, because they are powerless to single-handedly rid themselves of their addictions; (2) to complete a written list of all the people they have harmed with their tech addictions; and (3) to make restitution to those they have harmed.

The twelve-step protocol also advances a commitment by group members to believe that their lives will improve if their daily behaviors include honesty, hope, trust, truth, integrity, change of heart, humility, brotherly love, restitution and reconciliation, accountability, perseverance, and spirituality.

Finally, because members become part of the fellowship group to create *balance* in their lives and to help other tech users to achieve the same, the ITAA meetings routinely follow a prescribed agenda with these eleven parts: (1) check-in (includes announcements members want to share with fellow group members); (2) welcome by group leaders; (3) announcements by group leaders (such as ensuring that members turn off their tech gadgets before the meeting begins); (4) meeting (a reading of the twelve traditions and promises at the meeting's start); (5) visitors welcomed and invited to cite their first names, if they wish; (6) outline (the basic outline for the week's open discussion is read); (7) special topics (members encouraged to share their suggestions for particular topics of meeting focus); (8) basket passed (for those wanting to give financial contributions); (9) chips (i.e., tokens distributed to members for length of "tech sobriety"); (10) anonymity statements before the meeting's close (with expressions commonly including statements like, "Whom you see here and what you hear here is a *trust*, so let it stay here"); and (11) serenity prayer closing: "God, grant me the serenity to accept the things I cannot change, the courage to change the things I can, and the wisdom to know the difference."

47. What is Camp Grounded, who goes there, and why?

There is little question that in Silicon Valley, technologies take on an almost cult-like status, for newly created tech tools are broadly viewed as enabling incredible self-empowerment. The developers of these emerging technologies, in fact, often hope that their high-tech discoveries will provide them with the means for early financial freedom.

Also housed in California is Camp Grounded—a camp run by the Digital Detox Company. Created by the late Levi Felix and his close friends and family in 2013, the premise of Camp Grounded is to challenge not only the over-use of technology by individuals but the moral compass of technology companies. Today, Camp Grounded makes an annual call for high-tech users to temporarily reject their smartphones, computers, and digital watches—and join other camp attendees for a weekend's fun-filled, reflection period. Yearly, Camp Grounded allows grown-ups to congregate during the warmer months in the Mendocino National Forest, just north of San Francisco Bay. Digital devices are banned at the camp, as are participants' real names, work talk, alcohol, and drugs. For around $1,000, campers gather for four days and three nights to "unplug," get away, and, importantly, be free again, just as in childhood!

Who typically registers for the camp? Attendees are predominantly economically comfortable Americans who live and work in the Bay area. Age-wise, they are typically in their twenties and thirties, and there generally are more women than men attending. Most attendees are Caucasian, with Asians being the second-largest demographic, followed by Hispanics. Those residing outside the Bay area tend to be older and have families. Politically, attendees' views inform their strong feelings about the tech industry, their beliefs that natural or organic foods are the best consumable for the body, and their overall perception that Camp Grounded will provide great personal value for the money. In short, attendees seem to firmly believe that this four-day "natural existence" kind of connect with other attendees will be nourishing for their souls, primarily because that is how humans evolved. In fact, the basic premise behind Camp Grounded is that while "detoxing with food" aims to remove what is considered to be toxic to an individual's diet, "detoxing with digital devices" aims to remove what is considered to be toxic to an individual's life satisfaction and well-being.

What can attendees expect to do at Camp Grounded over the weekend? First, when they arrive, retreat organizers tell attendees that human contact is inherently healthy. So at this adult camp, hugging another person is promoted, because it offers a lot of immediate benefits—like getting a burst of oxytocin— which not only lowers stress levels but delays signs of aging if this practice is continued after the retreat. Second, "playful" lodging is assigned on arrival, such that attendees stay in small villages named after animals (like Bobcat and Squirrel). Third, Saturday night is designated as a "special event" period. During the daylight hours, attendees are instructed to wear white clothes while engaging in several hours of silence to reflect on their greatest fears in life—which they are instructed to write on a piece of paper. On Saturday night, attendees are encouraged to burn the paper in an emotional ritual to, literally, burn away those fears.

Over the entire weekend, attendees engage in a series of fun, kid-like activities based on these three ingredients: (1) interpersonal connections, (2) a reverence for nature, and (3) a celebration of face-to-face human experiences. In fact, a number of practices and activities at Camp Grounded have been appropriated from Eastern and New Age spiritual rituals—such as yoga, meditation, silent eating (so attendees can reflect), wearing white clothes, and burning away one's fears.

While tech usage is strictly prohibited, it does appear in more nostalgic and symbolic forms; for example, there are a number of wooden stands around the campsite serving as land-based "inboxes" for participants to leave paper notes and gifts for other attendees. These wooden box symbols also serve as a kind of "human search engine," such that participants can write a question on a piece of paper, drop it in the wooden box, and come back later to see if someone has answered it. Because land-based, non-tech creativity is strongly encouraged throughout the weekend, there are manual typewriters spread throughout the camp for creative pursuits, and singing or playing musical instruments to entertain others is always welcome.

So how do attendees benefit from participating? Testimonials of "very happy campers" are displayed on the company website. Participants consistently say that their lives were *transformed* by their personal experiences at Camp Grounded. They also state that the pamphlet titled, "A Guide to Bringing Balance Back to Your Everyday Life," which they receive at the end of the event, continues to provide them with useful tips during the workweek to not only maintain their balance and life satisfaction but increase them. Practical advice offered in the pamphlet includes activities such as (1) "Liking" someone in person rather than virtually, (2) eating meals without one's digital devices, (3) buying an alarm clock for the bedroom instead of using a smartphone to wake in the morning, and (4) minimizing "shexting" (i.e., using the bathroom while texting). Many participants note that they continue to have contact with other attendees after the camp ends, and in these follow-up face-to-face gatherings or communiqués, they continue to pair their camp animal names with their real names.

Given that participants seem to be quite fond of Camp Grounded, what do its critics say? Answer: that there are a number of other digital detox protocols that cost considerably less than Camp Grounded or are free of charge. Finally, what do the high-tech companies in Silicon Valley say about Camp Grounded? A spokesperson from *Google* once said that of 200 employees who attended the camp (at the company's expense), when they came back to work, they were not only refreshed and "reconnected," but they appeared even more committed to their work-based human connections than before attending. In short, it seems that corporate-sponsored spokespersons and the Camp Grounded participants forcefully maintain that the benefits of attending continue well after the weekend event is finished—which explains why many attendees return year after year.

48. Are structured digital detox programs like Camp Grounded or Digital Detox Holidays really effective at changing technology over-use?

There is little question that in Silicon Valley, Camp Grounded is a way for techies to become more mindful of their technology over-use and to fully connect with other attendees over a fun-filled weekend. Globally, another alternative for tethered online users is to take a digital detox holiday alone or with family or friends at a designated "mindful" and digital-free or digital-limited resort. Hospitality management experts define "digital-free tourism" (DFT) as tourism spaces where internet and mobile phone signals are absent, or where digital technology access is limited or intentionally controlled by the resorts.

Nowadays, wellness travel is booming. By the end of 2023, the Global Wellness Institute projects that the industry will be worth $815.5 billion. Because currently the boom is often driven by women in middle age, it is not surprising that the latest trend in DFT is what has been dubbed "the Menopause Vacation." Also, "black hole" resorts—forbidding the use of any form of technology while on-site (including tvs, smartphones, or the internet)—are becoming especially popular in the United Kingdom and the United States. Also, digital detox holidays are drawing more and more surf-and-sand-seeking tourists of all age groups to tropical destinations like the Maldives, St. Vincent, and Little Palm Island in Florida. Of course, the expectations for the desired degree of technology available at the resort while on holiday are quite variable from one tourist to another. While some tourists want some internet connection while on holiday, others don't want any at all.

To get a better sense of the different types of DFT-inclined tourists, in 2019 a research team led by Daisy Fan from Bournemouth University in the UK conducted an interesting study to delineate the profiles of travelers at the one end having a high need for online contact with others in their home destinations while on holiday, compared to those at the other end having a high need for face-to-face contact with others at their travel destinations. And what did the research team discover? That there are at least six different traveler profiles that DFT resorts should consider providing for.

Let's now look more closely at these six types. There are the (1) social media addicts, who maintain high levels of social media presence as a tourist—posting to those in their virtual orbit holiday scenery, holiday foods purchased, and people met; (2) daily life controllers (or so-called "responsibility" types), who like to maintain frequent virtual contact with their home social groups (particularly their children) while on holiday because of their stated commitments to "check-in regularly"; (3) dual zone travelers, who try to capitalize on both their online home social contacts and their face-to-face vacation contacts while on holiday; (4) diversionary travelers, uniquely both low online-contact-driven and low face-to-face contact-driven, who seem motivated by their need to relax, to recover, and to escape from their internet-connected daily life; (5) digital detox travelers, who mindfully reject their "home zones" to be fully engaged in the "away zone" by switching off their smartphones once onsite and not connecting to the internet until returning home; and (6) disconnected immersive travelers, who are all about having high face-to-face communications with the "away zone"—admitting that they don't even go online much at home because of privacy concerns and a preference for solid "old-fashioned" communication habits.

So now for the big question: Do Camp Grounded attendees and DFT travelers believe that these two types of "mindful breaks" from technology use have a positive impact on their well-being? Given the evidence collected to date, the bottom line seems to be this: That participants returning from digital detox resorts or Camp Grounded consistently say that taking even a short break from technology engagement not only provided them with the opportunity to refuel, relax, and "mindfully" reconnect with others on land—but reinforced the notion that routinely engaging in a digital detox is beneficial for the mind and the soul.

49. How do I find a therapist to help me create a better relationship with technology?

If you believe that you have a technology over-use problem and want to find a therapist to help you have a better relationship with technology, there are a number of options available to you. If you are a student, most schools and universities have a specially designated person or department to help you obtain access to a therapist. If you are employed full-time, a number of larger organizations have an Employee Assistance Program (EAP) in place that includes access to mental health experts. Given the many land-based and virtual-based therapy options available today, you will need to determine early on whether you prefer an online therapist or a land-based one so that a good fit can be found for you.

Before visiting a therapist, you may also want to inform yourself about what to expect during the sessions, and whether the time is right for you to see someone. Nowadays, there are a number of online therapy aids that may prove valuable information in this regard. For example, in 1995, Dr. John M. Grohol, a US psychologist, created the website PsychCentral—which still remains active. It describes in detail what is meant by Internet Addiction Disorder (IAD); provides a series of self-help tests, podcasts, and sample therapists' questions; and provides useful steps for finding a therapist or a support group in your area. The betterhelp website is another excellent source to help you locate a virtually based therapist with certain characteristics you are seeking.

What kind of therapeutic interventions can you expect from the therapist? The most used and arguably very successful treatment for various forms of online addiction is cognitive behavioral therapy (CBT). For example, at Dr. Kimberly Young's Center for Internet Addiction in the United States, CBT is used as a treatment tool for clients clinically assessed as suffering from internet addiction. In this treatment program, clients are taught to monitor their thoughts to identify likely provoking feelings and actions leading to their online addiction. Clients are also taught how to hone new coping skills and other means of "balancing" their land-based and virtually based life activities to prevent addiction relapses from occurring once the therapy sessions are completed. This Center's website also provides a useful Internet Addiction Test (IAT) that online users can complete in the privacy of their homes to ascertain whether they have a technology over-use problem that calls for a trained therapist's intervention.

CBT therapy generally requires weekly sessions of forty-five minutes or so with the mental health expert, with the typical duration period being three to four months. At the early stages of CBT, the therapy focuses on specific behaviors in life situations where a client's impulse control disorder causes the greatest difficulty in avoiding a need to go online. As the CBT sessions evolve, the focus tends to move to the cognitive (i.e., thought) assumptions and distortions that have become ingrained in the online user and that drives the need to go online. Therapists note, for example, that individuals suffering from a negative core of self-beliefs are often drawn to the anonymous interactive capabilities of the internet to either mediate or overcome their perceived personal shortcomings.

Besides CBT or Motivational Interviewing (where clients openly discuss with the therapist their personal goals desired post-treatment), other kinds of treatment protocols have been developed by mental health experts to help clients recover from particular kinds of online addictions. For example, a specialized and comprehensive treatment protocol for Internet Gaming Disorder (IGD) in adolescents and teens, called PIPATIC, was developed in 2018 by a research team led by Professor Alexandra Torres-Rodriguez. This special treatment program integrates several areas of a therapist's intervention into six modules (delivered over twenty sessions or less). The six modules include: (1) a psychoeducational therapy-focus; (2) a typical treatment therapy-focus (like CBT); (3) an intrapersonal therapy-focus; (4) an interpersonal-therapy focus; (5) a family intervention-therapy focus; and (6) a more "balanced" lifestyle-therapy focus. The long-term goals of PIPATIC therapy are to reduce the client's addiction symptoms related to online games and to improve the well-being of adolescents and teens. To accomplish these goals, the program is customized for each client. In data collected so far, the program appears to work well—with significant improvements reported by clients in key areas of life functioning and in their ability to maintain well-being over the longer term.

50. Can you complete a digital detox regimen by yourself? How?

There is nothing that stops individuals from completing a self-imposed digital detox. In fact, before starting therapy with a mental health expert, committing to complete a digital detox is often a requirement. Also, there are a number of "do it yourself" digital detox books on the market that you can read, including Blake Snow's 2017 book titled *Log Off: How to Stay Connected after Disconnecting*. In just a hundred pages, this lifestyle journalist shares his own experiences at undergoing self-imposed digital detoxes.

If you are considering starting your own digital detox regimen and you want some pointers from someone who is a "pro" at doing this, Blake Snow offers these five practical tips: (1) *remove distractions*: because family, friends, health, and work are important to our life satisfaction and well-being—anything not essential to these four "burners in life" should be removed, starting with your initial detox period; (2) *do not glamorize busyness*: by not glamorizing busyness, we can think about what the busyness is intended to replace in our lives and instead focus on how we can wisely spend precious time on land-based activities that better meet our personal needs, starting with the initial digital detox period; (3) *always ask "why?" when you feel the urge to pull out your smartphone*: instead of "pushing down" our anxiety when we are feeling alone or accessing social media sites to hear what our friends are doing, we should consciously choose *not* to use our smartphones as an emotional security blanket, particularly during this digital detox period; by doing so, we can remember how to not only "be present in the moment" but be grateful for that moment; (4) *try using the rule of thirds*: to optimize our happiness and productivity, we need to ensure that our lives routinely include eight hours for work or school activities, eight hours for sleep, and eight hours of free time to let our minds wander or to engage in land-based activities that we find truly enjoyable—so begin to accomplish this rule during the digital detox period; and (5) *periodically—and beginning with this digital detox period, literally fast from your digital toys*: after this initial digital detox trial, take a week each spring and fall, say, with no connection to the internet to mindfully connect with others we truly care for and to mindfully connect with ourselves.

Dr. Pathak, an academic counselor at Indira Gandhi National Open University in India, adds to Snow's list of pointers. He suggests that before committing to do a digital detox, you should make two lists. First, list all of your digital gadgets to show you how dependent you have become on technology. Second, make a list of all the things you enjoy doing in life but are not presently doing because of being too engaged with your tech devices. If the second list is compelling, you have just gained insight that by reducing your technology use, you will regain some precious time to do the land-based things you really enjoy but have dismissed.

Also, warns Dr. Pathak, failed digital detoxes are often the result of overwhelming ourselves with unachievable targets. So pick some part of your daily routine when you can omit engaging with technology—maybe on your lunch break, when exercising, or when out shopping. By slowly eliminating technology from part of your day, you will make it easier on yourself to stay the full course of a longer digital detox. Finally, find a digital detox buddy. Because a support system is always good to have when doing a digital detox, both of you can discuss your progress, encourage each other to continue with the digital detox for a longer period, and spend "mindful" time with each other face-to-face rather than by text-messaging. In short, a digital detox buddy will help keep you honest and fully committed to the process.

51. Is regularly unplugging for, say, a religious Shabbat a form of digital detox?

Yes, regularly unplugging for a religious Shabbat is a form of digital detox. While undergoing a digital detox typically means refraining from using online devices for a certain length of time, the detox period may also include refraining from using other more conventional items like televisions or work-related tools and programs. These restrictions apply to individuals regularly "unplugging" for the twenty-five hours of Shabbat—a practice that has existed in the observant Jewish community for centuries, where the use of electricity by community members is strictly forbidden on the weekly day of rest known as Shabbat. This law was derived from the saying, "You shall not kindle fire in any of your dwellings on Sabbath day."

What benefits do those committed to unplugging for the twenty-five hours of Shabbat on a weekly basis say they gain? In an interesting 2016 study completed by Irene Michaels, a registered nurse, holistic health practitioner, and graduate student at St. Catherine's University in Minnesota, she interviewed at length six individuals who engaged in Shabbat to understand their perceived holistic health benefits—physical, mental, and spiritual.

Seven beneficial themes surfaced through discussions with the participants and through their visual images shared as representing their "mindful" Shabbat periods: (1) *mental relief*: the participants experienced a strong feeling of peace and serenity—such that being unplugged for Shabbat was like "a spa for your brain"; (2) *social connection*: the participants enjoyed the meals they had with friends and family—and, they emphasized, at the Shabbat lunch, everyone stayed until late in the relaxing afternoon, in contrast to during the week when no one is relaxed and is constantly checking the smartphone; (3) *self-care*: the participants completed fulfilling, self-relaxing activities not doable during the week—such as time alone to take a walk, read, nap, or just think; (4) *nature*: the participants took time to connect with the world in a different way, "in a nature sense," by the lake, in the forest, or at the beach; (5) *spiritual community*: the participants attended the synagogue—leaving them feeling "connected" to their community, to their friends, and to God—a real communal experience; (6) *stress*: the participants said that while being unplugged during Shabbat was frustrating or irritating at times because they realized that there was only one day left on the weekend to get stuff done, they were definitely not ready to stop the observance or the unplugging; and (7) *spirituality*: the participants consistently remarked that they had "a spiritual reawakening" by unplugging for the Shabbat—like "a breath of fresh air," "like another Shabbat soul was joining mine," or "like experiencing a taste of heaven."

52. Is it possible to receive online help from an expert so I can better manage my technology use?

Yes, it is possible to receive online help from a mental health expert so you can learn to better manage your technology use if you choose to go that route. Broadly speaking, internet addiction therapy aims to help an individual moderate internet use to not only cope with this psychological dependency but to heal from the negative mental, physical, and relationship effects generated by online over-use. As with land-based therapy sessions, online interventions designed by mental health professionals tend to incorporate various forms of talk therapy—such as cognitive behavioral therapy (CBT), interpersonal therapy, motivational interviewing (to help clients explore discrepancies between their current state and their desired mental and physical health state), and group therapy (i.e., undergoing treatment sessions with others experiencing similar issues).

The goal of talk therapy—whether it is delivered on land or online—is to help the technology over-user to change their beliefs, to understand their triggers for incessantly going online, to improve their land-based interpersonal functioning, and to find support and alternative fulfilling life activities. As in land-based therapy sessions, treatment options suggested by online mental health experts—with the client's acceptance—are typically customized to the individual's personal factors or stated preferences.

Is online mental health counseling effective in assisting clients to overcome their online dependency? In recent years, notes psychiatrist Dr. Elias

Aboujaoude from Stanford University, the telepsychiatry platform revolution, per se—defined as the technology-mediated delivery of mental health care—has been evolving rapidly. It has brought into the mental health sphere computerized CBT, online video-based therapy, enhanced efficiency, reduced stigma associated with visiting land-based mental health clinics, and the ability for clients to bypass diagnosis-specific obstacles to their treatment. For example, clients suffering from social anxiety often are not willing to leave the comfort of their homes, so online therapy is useful.

Having said this, Dr. Aboujaoude adds that there is continued resistance by some clients to go the online therapy route. For example, some clients are concerned about their privacy invasion if they obtain their therapy online. Other clients say they want to try some high-tech apps for weaning themselves from their digital devices instead, but most of these apps have not undergone controlled effectiveness assessments by their developers, so it seems premature at this stage to confirm that they are clinically effective. Finally, though the present-day reality is that more clients seem to gravitate toward land-based therapy sessions (even after the Covid-19 lockdowns), it seems totally reasonable that in the near future, a "click here if you are addicted to the internet" approach might prove to be an equally sought after strategy for helping addicts to break free from their compulsive online behaviors.

53. What are some technology-based tools or apps that can help you limit your screen time, online gaming, or social media use?

Smartphones have a number of built-in features to help you cut back on your screen time. These include using the grayscale functionality to not only save the battery's power but make attention-getting bright app icons less obvious. You can also disable notifications or badges to alleviate attention-demanding alerts. Here are five other smartphone features and pointers for reducing your screen time: (1) *home screen*: limit your tools to only necessary ones (e.g., maps, calendar) to reduce your time spent on other apps; (2) *audio messaging*: use this messaging tool rather than the text messaging one to reduce your time spent on your device; (3) *social media apps*: delete your social media apps from your phone and commit to only using them while you are on your computer; (4) *phone alarm*: do not use your smartphone alarm at bedtime but rely on a conventional alarm clock to encourage a more enduring and refueling sleep; and

(5) *night shift*: use this feature to reduce your exposure to blue light—known to disrupt a sound night's sleep.

Adding to these built-in smartphone features are a number of new and inexpensive high-tech products designed with particular objectives in mind to help you minimize your screen time and to optimize your well-being. Here are nine popular apps, along with portions of the taglines used for their marketing purposes: (1) *Flipd*: locks you out of your nonessential phone functions so you can focus on your school or work activities, engage in a wellness hub, or train your brain to refocus—tagline is "Time is precious—*Flipd* helps you spend it well"; (2) *Thrive*: limits your interactions with those not on your "Favorites" list, disables problematic apps at the preset threshold, and explains your lack of responses through the auto-reply feature—tagline is "The *Thrive* platform improves communication with frontline staff, builds a stronger team, creates a community, nurtures talent, shares successes, supports leadership"; (3) *Siempo*: replaces your home screen with less distracting interfaces, un-brands icons, batches notifications, and separates essential tools from other apps—tagline is "Use your tech, not the other way around"; (4) *Freedom*: blocks sites deemed to be problematic for you and is designed to keep you off your phone for eight hours at a time—tagline is "Used by over 1,000,000 people to reclaim focus and productivity"; (5) *RescueTime*: blocks sites deemed to be problematic for you—tagline is "Take back control of your time"; (6) *uBlock Origin*: blocks sites seemed to be problematic for you, particularly third-party ads, trackers, and malware—tagline is "You decide what enters your browser"; (7) *F.lux*: reduces your exposure to sleep-disrupting blue light—tagline is "It makes the color of your computer's display adapt to the time of day, warm at night, and like the sunlight during the day"; (8) *Space*: designed to help you think about how you use your phone and how it negatively affects your life—tagline is "Find your phone/life balance"; and (9) *SelfControl*: lets you block your own access to distracting websites, mail servers, or anything else on the internet—tagline is "A free Mac application to help you avoid distracting websites."

On a closing cautionary note, mental health experts say that while it is unlikely that any of these apps, software add-ons, or program extensions is "unsafe" for users, there is a tendency for the providers to market these without sufficient testing for clinical effectiveness. If users are seriously concerned that they may have an internet addiction problem, they should seek an evaluation and treatment by a qualified mental health expert in favor of just using one or more of these digital device apps.

54. How can I get off my phone and be more present when I'm in social situations?

Let's face it, "phubbing" someone in front of you by texting on your phone instead of mindfully engaging in conversation with that person is downright rude. So how can you become less connected to your phone and more present when you're in social situations? Let's ask some experts.

First, to overcome separation anxiety from your smartphone—known as nomophobia—Dr. Marlynn Wei, a board-certified Harvard- and Yale-trained psychiatrist, advises clients to weaken the action-reward link by sitting without access to their phones while it charges, and then increasing the no-access period of time day after day. The whole point of this exercise, she says, is to show you that you will survive without constant access to your smartphone. Other tactics include meditating in the morning instead of checking your smartphone messages first thing; deferring checking your phone further into the morning by reading, drawing, or doing some other land-based activity; and handwriting a letter to someone you are thinking about rather than sending this person an email or text message on your phone. Also, regularly schedule more land-based connection time with your family and friends by routinely letting your smartphone battery drain to zero.

But, you may wonder, are these suggestions realistic for young adults who are digital natives—literally, born with a digital device in their hands? In an interesting 2018 study conducted by graduate students Linda Miksch and Charlotte Schultz at Lund University in Sweden, the researchers conducted in-depth interviews with twelve young adults from eight countries (Switzerland, Germany, China, Turkey, the United States, Finland, and Canada) who said they were actively implementing strategies in their lives to reduce their digital interactions and to increase their land-based "connectedness" with others.

What were their motivations for doing so? Their stated motivations for making this lifestyle change included: (1) maintaining more self-control instead of succumbing to their fear of missing out (FOMO) on friends' news—and constantly checking the smartphone; (2) increasing their productivity at work or school instead of surfing online for topics of interest; (3) improving their well-being by making a conscientious effort to stop using social media to communicate with friends or coworkers and to build a toolbox that includes more nostalgic forms of communicating; (4) being "in the moment" by spending more time with friends and family to have "real" conversations with them instead of sending them short text messages on the smartphone; and

(5) maintaining solid relationships with family and friends by dialoging more openly and honestly with them rather than half-listening while attending to messages on the smartphone (i.e., phubbing them).

What strategies did these young adults use to accomplish their objectives? Here are three cognitive strategies that they relied on: (1) in the professional environment, took actions such as creating a greater self-awareness to set clear work-life priorities, made use of personal rules for maintaining work-life balance, and actively created self-pressure—including setting up physical barriers to prevent excessive interactions with their digital technology; (2) in the private environment, took actions such as using self-reflective strategies for not only continually being aware of a potential digital device over-use problem but exercising self-control by making "mindful choices" to maintain a work-life balance—like not being physically, visibly, or functionally available to outside demands by others and leaving digital devices behind when exercising or doing other fun life activities; and (3) in the social environment, took actions such as creating barriers to prevent interaction with digital technologies, both self-imposed and group-imposed—including agreeing with friends and family to connect through one phone call or, preferably, through face-to-face meetings instead of using multiple text messages or emails.

The researchers concluded that these study findings suggest the need for digital natives to shift back in time and to regularly disconnect from technology to become more "authentic in the moment." Without question, the interviewees perceived the topic of "digital detox" to be extremely personal, emotional, and sensitive, indicating that they perceived real harms from past heavy tech usage and didn't want to keep going back there.

55. Is "quiet quitting" a form of digital detox?

If you are a *TikTok* aficionado, you probably first heard of "quiet quitting" in July 2022, when a user named "zaidleppelin" got millions of views on a video he posted on this topic. What exactly is quiet quitting, and is it a form of digital detox? The video explained why many Generation Z employees (those born between 1997 and 2012) refuse to "burn themselves out" over their jobs, so they are increasingly turning to another lifestyle for a more balanced mode of operating. In fact, the new norm they are advocating is closer to "quiet quitting," but the exact definition of what this entails is still evolving. Perhaps it is safe to say that "quiet quitting" is doing the opposite of working hard for someone else. Instead, energy is saved to keep one's own life balanced.

Seen in a positive light, "quiet quitting" is not actually quitting your job but focusing on your life outside of your job. This may mean not taking on weekend work if you'd rather have fun with friends and family or refusing to stay beyond a meeting's pre-set curtain fall. Some more extremists may decide to work as little as possible but still meet the employer's expectations in order to be paid. (You may have heard about soon-to-be-retirees who really don't love their jobs and choose to become quiet quitters until the big send-off day.)

Perhaps the turning point for Gen Z young adults came at the time of the Covid-19 pandemic, when they were tethered to their computers for school or work. If they worked, it was probably in the fast food industry—where the risks for getting the virus were high (because no vaccines had yet been developed) and where their wages were low. Being tech-savvy, they understood that work or school assignments could be done in a variety of ways—including via a hybrid land-based/virtual approach. There is little question that the "quiet quitting" video may have tapped into a new "digital detox" kind of thinking and behaving—especially for people in this age group, who moving forward will be integral in defining the evolving landscape of work-life balance.

56. How do you establish better work-life boundaries to reduce the amount of time you spend "plugged in" to work after hours?

We live in a hyper-connected world. With this reality, far too many companies globally feel that they can freely access their employees—and have them quickly respond—seven days a week for 365 days a year because of the internet, smartphone text messaging, and company email. But this presumption by industry has mental health experts like Cary Cooper of the University of Manchester in the United Kingdom worried, because unlimited access can not only cause digital exhaustion in employees—thus adversely impacting their work and home productivity levels—but contribute to their "presenteeism." That is, when employees go to work ill so they can physically be present, they tend not to produce much in terms of real value, often because of lack of quality sleep and much-needed time to refuel. Professor Cooper says that this long working-day syndrome, combined with digital device over-use, creates tremendous stress, anxiety, and depression in employees, leading far too often to physician-prescribed stress leaves.

So how can employees establish better work-life boundaries to reduce the amount of time they spend "plugged in" to work after hours? First, jurisdictions around the world (including Italy, the Netherlands, Belgium, Canada, and Kenya) have increasingly jumped on the pass legislation bandwagon to create a clearer work-life boundary for employees. For example, in August 2016, France adopted the El Khomri law, or *loi Travail*, offering French employees the right to "disconnect" from work calls and emails during nonworking hours. Under this first-to-be passed "right to disconnect law," companies having more than fifty people are obliged to create a charter of good conduct to set out the hours—normally in the evenings and on the weekends—when staff are not supposed to send or answer work-related emails. What sanctions are imposed for companies found not to be compliant? In July 2018, as a case in point, France's Supreme Court ordered *Rentokil Initial*, a British pest control company, to pay 60,000 Euros (about $65,000) to a former employee required by the company to be constantly accessible.

As for employees themselves setting some work-life boundaries, many have chosen to turn on the "silence notifications" option on their smartphones after a certain hour (say, 9:00 p.m.) and/or employing the "out of office" flag on their email (say, on the weekends). Or they set up assertive auto-responses and signature lines to dissuade off-the-clock work communications from others—such as, "I'm sending this email at a time that works for me, so please only reply at a time that works for you." Colleagues at work quickly get the message that this employee has set a clear work-life boundary when it comes to acceptable digital access beyond a certain hour of the day or certain days of the week. This boundary-setting exercise also sends the subtle message to colleagues that, "I'm doing high-quality work in the hours that I have."

57. What work-life balance and well-being maintenance lessons were learned during the Covid-19 pandemic lockdowns, and how can they be helpful in the future?

When Covid-19 struck, students and working adults, alike, were greatly impacted. Besides being afraid to catch the virus—as there were no vaccines yet available, individuals of all ages were tethered to their computers to complete school and work assignments, Mental health and business experts now report that there were a number of key work-life balance and well-being maintenance lessons learned during the lockdown periods that can be helpful now and in the future. Let's look more closely at five of these critical ones.

First, claiming "me time" without guilt is necessary to maintain our mental and physical health by setting boundaries between work/school parts of the day and leisure or refueling parts of the day and night. Without question, the benefits of routinely disconnecting from digital devices are myriad—including improving our creativity and productivity, maintaining our land-based relationships (as well as the virtual ones), and sustaining our work-life balance and quality of life over the longer term.

Second, getting a sound sleep nightly without any interruptions/blue light emissions from our smartphones is critical. Simply put, our brains need recharging away from school or work, and bedtime is the way we were designed by nature to "refuel." If our brains ruminate on negative and stressful things before bedtime, it will do so much longer than if the rumination period is on positive thoughts. So, if we're answering arousing emails or text messages until we turn off the lights (or even after), our brains don't have enough time to shut down properly or effectively heal overnight. Consequently, exhaustion lingers into the morning.

Third, the new boundary-setting protocol around "on" and "off" hours applies as well to our relationships. For many families during the two-year lockdown, parents, their kids, and even their pets shared their home's physical and virtual spaces. Post-pandemic, many adults have said that they reached insight about how terribly over-subscribed and stressed-out they were not only because of this communal sharing of space but because of the quickly changed life roles they were expected to play—often as teacher, caregiver, and employee. When the pandemic ended, many adults affirmed that they've now moved toward an energy "rebalancing act," brought on by reflections gained during this stressful period. Simply put, they affirm, that there need to be honest conversations within the family around the importance of relationship boundaries and each individual's role within this dynamic.

Fourth, the good news is that remote work practices and technologies, hurriedly deployed during the pandemic lockdowns, proved broadly successful—even on a global scale. To the dismay of many employers finding themselves still paying for costly office lease space post-pandemic, many remote workers now strongly prefer to keep working from home, because they say they were less stressed and had improved well-being (and safety) by doing so. In fact, in a May 2023 survey distributed to 5,800 remote workers conducted by Canadian researchers Graham Lowe, Karen Hughes, and Jim Stanford, 40 percent of those surveyed said that they want to work from home *all the time*, and another 56 percent said they want to continue doing so *most or some of the time.* That means only 4 percent of remote workers prefer returning to regular workplaces full-time! These study results underscore the importance of employers' having meaningful conversations and negotiations with employees and their unions about future remote-work arrangements. No one knows how remote work will evolve over the longer term, but thanks to the pandemic, it's clearly here to stay.

Fifth, from an employer point of view, the two-year lockdowns undoubtedly led to mental health struggles among small business owners, in particular. Calling it a mental health "echo pandemic," the Ontario Chamber of Commerce reported in October 2023, that of 60,000 small business owners contacted by them, 45 percent said that they felt "overwhelming stress" dealing with the effects of the pandemic—exacerbated by inflation, supply chain issues, and employee retention. In fact, 67 percent of them said they either were "burnt out" or close to it after two years of stress—leaving them in a state of mental, emotional, and physical exhaustion day after day. Coupled with this finding is the present-day reality that they are now facing increased demands by employees for a wide range of mental health supports. The Chamber of Commerce is advocating for governments in Canada and elsewhere to consider offering tax incentives in the near future to encourage small business spending on employer and employee mental health initiatives—citing the impressive tax incentives offered in the United States via the Small Business Health Care Tax Credit.

Case Studies

Case 1. Barbara's Time Online Is Hurting Her Mental Health

Compared to many of her friends, Barbara was a previously non-tech-savvy teen who preferred playing sports and hanging out with friends at the mall or in the field. But she became a technology user once her family bought a home computer and loaded it with various apps and fun online games. Not too long after the computer arrived, Barbara developed an increased urge to check her emails and connect with friends on various social media platforms. She especially found *TikTok* to be a fun platform, because her friends posted some really funny videos of themselves doing wild dances or singing witty songs. The down side of being on these platforms, Barbara mused, is that she used to be proud of her athletic body, but some of the things she saw there made her start to feel bad about how her own body looked.

Barbara said to herself: "In this era of *Tumblr* thigh gaps and *Pinterest* flat-tummy posts, I think that my athletic body build is simply not appealing! Maybe I need to get started on reworking it so that my friends still think I'm attractive and great to hang-out with!"

In an effort to recreate her body image, Barbara found herself routinely saving, screen-shotting, and reading "get slim" body posts. She even started making the so-called "flat tummy drink recipe" she found online before heading out to school daily. Barbara tried convincing herself that the flat tummy drink was actually quite tasty, but it actually was very nasty.

Barbara's mother became concerned when she noticed a number of changes in her daughter's life routine, especially her recent fixation on her body image.

She said to her daughter, "Barbara, is there something wrong that you want to talk about? Ever since we got our computer, I've noticed that you've lost your interest in sports. Not only that, but you seem to be spending a lot of time communicating with your friends in social media rather than meeting them at the mall or in the sports field."

Barbara replied, "Mom, to be honest, I think the time has come for me to withdraw from my sports team to focus more on obtaining a nicer body. After all, some of my friends have told me that they are either contemplating or are already doing the same thing! Would you be okay with this?"

Her mom blurted out, "No, dear, this really worries me. Can I help you find a professional or school counselor so you can talk more openly about this? I'm concerned it's just not a healthy move for you or your friends."

Analysis

In April 2023, a bipartisan set of US lawmakers sharpened their sticks against *TikTok*, in particular, out of a fear that this social media platform is actually a Chinese government spying machine. But according to mental health experts, there are a lot of other good reasons this platform and others like it should be closely monitored or even deleted from teens' lives. Female teens, more than any other age group, seem to have a love-hate relationship with social media platforms. While teens like Barbara may quietly fear that they spend far too much time on social media—and are strongly influenced by what they see there, their fear of missing out (FOMO) on someone's cute video, say, is too strong a drive to resist! What's worse, not engaging with friends in social media means risking rejection by friends and, consequently, "social suicide."

According to UK mental health experts Daria Kuss and Mark Griffiths, Barbara is not alone in her newly acquired fixation on her body image. She is spending considerable time on social media sites and seems to be affected by celebrity "influencers" who appear to have the "perfect body." She is starting to believe that her body falls far short of this standard. The present-day reality, say these two mental health experts, is that teen females, compared to teen males, are more likely to fall victim to social media over-use, eating disorders, and online addiction, because they more often "virtually" connect with their peers through social media.

Like Barbara, female teens are motivated by a fear of missing out on their friends' activities. In fact, some would argue that Barbara is rapidly becoming part of a social media cult prevalent among teens and worrisome to her mother. In fact, recent 2023 stats released by Wallaroo Media show that 60 percent of the billion or so *TikTok* devotees, in particular, are under age thirty—with some as young as age ten. In fact, on average, teen *TikTok* users say that they open the app at least eight times a day, with 80 percent of them (again, mostly females) admitting to posting their own videos on the platform showing them "at their best."

What's more, while teen females are socially active on these social media platforms, warn mental health experts Kuss and Griffiths, they are being bombarded with ads promoting products for improving their body image— because that is how these companies make their profits. Unfortunately, social media over-usage in teen females, coupled with targeted advertising for this "attractive-focused" market, often results in their developing eating disorders and shopping addictions over the longer term.

So what advice would mental health experts have for Barbara at this stage? As her mother suggested, she would be well advised to speak to a high school counselor about her body image concerns and her fear of missing out on friends' fun times to help her maintain her mental and physical well-being in the long run. A mental health professional could help Barbara explore more fully whether she should retain or regain her previous interest in land-based sports rather than spend so much of her time in the virtual world—and being negatively impacted by it.

Case 2. Bob and His School Are Targets of a Ransomware Attack

It was a warm September day and school was back in session—virtually, that is. Because of a lockdown caused by the Covid-19 pandemic, Bob's high school superintendent transferred about 6,000 students and their teachers to the online classroom environment. The high school's IT department assured everyone that things were in order and that the school's network was safe and secure. The IT staff also asked the students and staff to be sure that the anti-virus software on their home computers was installed and up-to-date. Bob made sure that he followed these instructions.

Before turning on his computer to attend his first class on Monday morning, Bob got an unexpected text message from his friend Tom. The message said:

Hey, Bob, you'll never believe what I just saw! When I went on my favorite social media site to start my day off right, I saw an amazing video that opened with an animated short of a flaming motorcycle. But that's not all I saw. This animation was followed by a solid 50 minutes of screengrabs that shocked me and would probably shock you! Among the screengrabs were allegations of teacher abuse at our school, page after page of our fellow students' academic records, and—get ready for this, Bob—your mental health records that your doctor shared with the school.

Bob immediately responded, "Hey, dude, tell me this is the truth and that you're not 'pulling my leg!'"

Tom texted back, "Trust me, Bob. This is true!"

Bob left his bedroom and ran to the kitchen to tell his parents what Tom had just shared. Visibly shaken by this news, Bob's father immediately called the school to ask how this privacy invasion and online exposure of his son's medical records occurred. The school secretary picked up the call and immediately connected Bob's father to the principal's office.

Principal Jones listened while Bob's father shared his major concerns about the purported invasion of his son's privacy by someone's posting Bob's medical health records online that were previously shared in confidence with the school's administration. Principal Jones apologized for this incident and then said:

> Let me be transparent with you, sir. The school district's network has been hit with a ransomware attack. Some cybercriminals broke into our protected network, took sensitive data of our students and staff, and said that they encrypted the data. The bottom line is that we cannot access this critical data unless we supposedly agree to pay the bad buys a sizable ransom to get the decryption key from them. We've called in the authorities and some highly capable cyber security experts to get sound advice on how best to handle this serious problem. The hackers posted in their ransomware note to us that they will send us a decryptor key and return the data if we or our insurance company pays the demanded ransom *promptly* and using bitcoin—I guess so the money trail is hard to trace. But chances are we're not paying it, because we've been warned by the authorities that paying the ransom would be a bad move since it incentivizes criminals to continue with their exploits. I told the authorities that I was worried that the bad guys would follow through on their threat to release our students' and staff's very personal data to the public if they weren't paid by us. From what you are telling me, sir, they did just that, and your son's medical records are now available for the public to see online.

Bob's father responded, "Thanks for this update—though troubling it is. But how will my son's personally identifiable information be protected from more harm?"

Principal Jones replied, "Our students and staff will be offered identity theft protection services free of charge for a prescribed period, which we are still working out with the authorities and our cyber insurance company. Again, I am so sorry that your son's personal information has been publicly displayed because of this unforeseen hack attack." Bob's father was left wondering whether the school district's networks were adequately protected to prevent such a devastating attack.

Analysis

Clearly, Bob's school district is not alone as a ransomware attack victim. In the United States, alone, over 5 million students had their personal information exposed or leaked online in 2022–3, because their school's network was targeted by cyber criminals. Furthermore, at least 122 public school districts in the United States have been hit with ransomware exploits since 2021—with more than half resulting in the hackers' leaking sensitive school data online. Also, in a recent 2023 global survey completed by the cybersecurity company *Sophos*, 80 percent of school IT professionals reported being affected by ransomware attacks in the past year, some more seriously than others.

In the end and following updated advice from the authorities and the insurance company, Bob's school district did *not pay* the ransom demanded but relied on the cyber security consultants to help get the network back up and running and to restore files from "the cloud." As is also common following hack attacks (and consistent with what the principal told Bob's father), the affected students and staff were promptly advised in a letter prepared by lawyers working with the school district that they would be offered identity theft protection services free of charge for a prescribed period. However, the letter clearly stated that unfortunately it's impossible for the school to keep the stolen files from being publicly shared once they're posted online by the bad guys—often in social media platforms or in the Dark Web. Therefore, those individuals adversely impacted by the hack attack should continue to monitor their credit ratings and bank accounts for suspicious activities. If they spot anything questionable, they are well advised to contact the institution where the suspicious activity was thought to occur as well as the police.

As for Bob's father's concerns that the school district may have failed to secure its networks—thus making it vulnerable to a ransomware attack, cyber security experts warn that no matter how well prepared a company or institution thinks they are, being targeted for a costly exploit by very skilled hackers "is not a matter of if but when."

The devastating ransomware attack that struck the prominent casino chain MGM Resorts on September 11, 2023, serves as a recent example of such a surprise hack attack. In fact, this exploit had many experts questioning whether this company gambled with its customers' data by not installing the latest security protections. Over a ten-day period, everything from hotel room digital keys to slot machines wasn't working. Websites for many of MGM's properties went offline, and guests found themselves waiting for hours to check into the resort hotels or to get handwritten receipts for casino winnings. Some hotel guests' personal information was also stolen—including their names, contact information, gender, date of birth, driver's license or passport numbers, and Social Security Numbers.

After lengthy forensic investigations, it seems the attack started with a phone call—if reports citing the Scattered Spider ransomware hackers are to be believed. This ransomware gang is known to specialize in "social engineering" tactics— such that the cybercriminals manipulate victims into doing what they want or need by impersonating key people in the organization. In fact, this ransomware group is known to be especially skilled at "vishing," defined as gaining illegal access to systems via a "convincing" and "urgent" telephone call rather than using phishing (done via email).

The key takeaway is that the attacks on MGM Resorts indicate that even organizations you would think have the best cyber security protections in place are still vulnerable if skilled hackers like Scattered Spider use the right attack vector to obtain illegal access to the system. More often than not, posit cyber security experts, the most vulnerable attack vector is the weakest link in the system: a gullible and trusting human being who falls for the hackers' prank.

Case 3. Jeff Experiences "Sextortion" Online

Jeff installed the latest virus and malware protection software on his computer, feeling confident that he had taken the appropriate actions to stay safe while online. Given that he was keenly interested in communicating with his friends online, Jeff decided he would join a mobile phone social connection platform. But which one?

Jeff did considerable research to try to figure out which one to join. He said to his friend Sally, "Many of these smartphone platforms want me to share my smartphone number with them—and that really bothers me, because I don't want to be bombarded by phishing emails or other obnoxious intrusions. Plus, I see it as a violation of my privacy!" Sally asked Jeff, "What about *WhatsApp?* That one's very popular."

Jeff chuckled and then replied, "Sally, that provider is one of the culprits! So I've decided I'm probably going to join *Kik Messenger*, because it is one of a few providers not having the number-sharing requirement."

Jeff did as he shared with Sally, but before too long, he started getting disturbing online communications from someone on *Kik*, who wanted him to send nude photos of himself and engage in some rather distasteful sexual acts. Jeff said to himself, "How can I protect myself and stop whoever is sending me these awful requests?"

Humiliated by these ongoing requests from some mystery person and unable to tell his parents what he was experiencing because he was so embarassed, Jeff decided to contact the authorities. After they conducted some cyber forensics, the police discovered that the person sending these disturbing requests to him was Jeff's former junior high school teacher. Jeff was also told by the police that he was not the only young person receiving these disturbing requests. Apparently his teacher used *Kik* to groom at least four other male teens who had also been former students, urging them to send sexual photos of themselves and to take part in various sexual acts. Sadly, some of them did—and over a considerable period of time. "So what's going to happen now?" Jeff asked.

The officer reassured him, "The teacher has been charged of a criminal offense involving obscene acts with minors in the virtual space. We generally regard this kind of activity as child luring—whether it occurs on land or online. It is considered to be a heinous act worthy of severe punishment by society's standards."

Jeff waited patiently for this case to come to trial. He was relieved when he learned that the former teacher was found to be guilty of the charges. The perpetrator was sanctioned by the judge and sent to federal prison for sixty years.

Analysis

What Jeff and the other male teens experienced is called, as the officer described, "online luring." Other charges involved often include "sextortion," particularly if the perpetrator of the crime threatens to disseminate the sexually revealing photos provided by the victims to friends, parents, or teachers if the victims fail to pay the demanded funds or fails to meet other demands. In democratic jurisdictions like the United States and Canada, online luring is viewed as a criminal offense involving the use of technology—such as texting, email messaging, or chatting in an app/game/website—to communicate with minors, with the intent of committing a sexual offense against them.

The perpetrator in these cases, typically an adult, uses a variety of tactics to "groom" the targets—including sending them sexually arousing material, misrepresenting who they really are (often saying that they are a teen of similar age), or attempting to establish a romantic relationship. The perpetrator's end goal—which commonly begins rather low key and then builds with intensity and offensiveness over time, is that the minor will either meet the offender in person and/or deliver the demanded sexually explicit material online. If the minor fails to deliver the photos or wants to end the virtual relationship, the perpetrator will often resort to blackmail or extortion.

Sadly, as far too many recent child luring cases have shown, the young victims often feel that the only way to end the torture and humiliation is through drug-induced escapes or suicide attempts. A recent case detailed by the media involved a twelve-year-old British Columbia (BC) Canadian male who died of a self-inflicted gunshot wound on October 12, 2023, following an apparent case of online sextortion. While the authorities are actively trying to determine who the perpetrator is, they affirm that the crime of sextortion seems to be on the rise in Canada as well as globally, in large part because so many teens are active on social media platforms and are overly trusting of strangers.

Following this death, the British Columbia Attorney General posited that unfortunately minors seem to feel that they need to suffer alone, but those experiencing this horror are well advised to share what is going on with a trusted adult so that authorities can be brought in to investigate the matter. In fact, in the jurisdiction where this young male was victimized, the authorities note that the targets' ages tend to be in the 13–18 range and involve both male and female targets. In just one year, the number of online child luring and sextortion cases investigated in this BC jurisdiction, alone, climbed from fifty-six to sixty-two.

Jeff was smart to contact the authorities regarding the online abuse he was experiencing so that they could intervene. In Canada, for example, the sanctions imposed by the courts on criminals found guilty of online luring, harassing, stalking, and extortion range from a summary offense (which is less serious) to an indictable offense (which is very serious and involves significant time behind bars). The judge hearing the evidence follows sentencing guidelines for that jurisdiction, adjusting the sanctions imposed on the criminal by the degree of harm experienced by the victim(s).

Notably, in November 2023, though the Supreme Court of Canada struck down a minimum one-year mandatory penalty for adults using the internet to lure minors into sexual activity but held that in Canada, judges should be tougher in sentencing the guilty perpetrators than they had been in the past. Why? Because the tremendous psychological damage these acts cause victims is more clearly understood.

Investigators advise that anyone who believes they are a victim of child luring or sextortion should immediately stop all communication with the perpetrator and not give in to their demands. Victims are also advised to deactivate any online accounts used to communicate with the perpetrator and immediately report the activity to trusted caregivers and the police.

Case 4. Ben Is Addicted to Online Games

Ben, a seventeen-year-old high school student, lives with his single mother, who is having financial struggles keeping them housed and fed, though she is working two jobs.

"Ben," his mother said, "I need you to get a part-time job to help us 'make ends meet.' And while we're discussing much needed changes, I also want you to focus more on your school work instead of playing online games for hours on end with your buddies, particularly well into the night when you should be sleeping!"

Ben's mom became very upset when shortly after this honest conversation, she found Ben "passed out" in front of his computer when he had school the next day.

"What's going on, Ben?" she asked.

Ben replied,

> Mom, I'm embarrassed you found me sleeping in front of my computer screen instead of being in bed, but I must confess that I played well into the night to optimize my game-playing 'high.' Oh, and Mom, I've got more to tell you. Now, don't be mad, but I've been using methamphetamines so I can continue playing up to 32 hours at a time. To be honest, no matter how hard I try, I just can't stop my urge to play!

After taking a deep sigh, his mom responded,

> Ben, this really worries me, because you have a medical history of obsessive behavior and depression. Maybe you should consider registering with an affordable self-help group like the Internet and Tech Addicts Anonymous, or ITAA. I understand from other parents that it is a free fellowship group meant

to help people of all ages trying to curb their technology over-use and addiction issues. While I'd like to send you to the digital detox Camp Grounded, Ben, where a couple of your school friends had gone and found it to be very therapeutic and fun, we are really short of money. I just don't see that as a real option for us at this point in time.

Ben said,

Mom, your concerns and advice seem totally justified. As I've shared with you already, I've tried stopping my intense game play at night, but I just can't fix it alone. Let me look into what that ITAA is all about. Maybe I can talk to a counselor at school about some other options that may be able to help me and not cost you a bundle.

Analysis

Ben's and his mom's concerns seem warranted, as he appears to be spending an excessive amount of time in online game play. He may even be an active online gamer during the daytime when he should be studying at school but is either in denial or reluctant to share this reality with his mom.

Experts may even suggest that Ben is or could eventually be clinically assessed as being online gaming-disordered, if not addicted. From a medical perspective, Internet Gaming Disorder (IGD), better known as gaming addiction, is defined by mental health experts as the pathological playing of video games, resulting in significant mental and/or behavioral harms to the player.

There is little question that after Ben agrees to be clinically assessed, a mental health expert would tell Ben's mother that she has a right to be concerned about his well-being in the present and over the longer term—especially since he has a medical history of obsessive behavior and depression. Ben's recent confession that he has started using methamphetamines to be able to play longer, especially at night, is an added point of concern.

Dr. Ashley Voss of the Naval Medical Center San Diego in the United States affirms that game-addicted individuals often manifest psychological triggers, cravings, and addiction-seeking behaviors typically found in alcoholics or substance addicts. Also, it is not uncommon for other kinds of addictive behaviors to be co-occurring with online game addiction, including alcohol or drug abuse, obsessive pornography engagement, anxiety, depression, attention-deficit/hyperactivity disorder (ADHD), and various other personality disorders. Therefore, as Ben has admitted, he and fellow gaming addicts would have difficulty overcoming these well-being threats alone. They would benefit greatly from therapeutic interventions under the care of a mental health expert specializing in this field.

Though Camp Grounded was one option discussed by Ben and his mother, this therapeutic activity is typically meant for individuals less addicted to technology. In the end, the mental health provider assessing Ben's condition may suggest that he not only undergo psychological treatment for his IGD but also consider joining an addiction fellowship group like Internet and Tech Addicts Anonymous for added peer support.

So how prevalent is IGD in the general population, you may wonder? In 2020, a research team led by Nazia Darvesh, affiliated with St. Michael's Hospital in Toronto, Canada, tried to answer this question. The researchers reviewed 160 published studies using thirty-five different methods to diagnose IGD and its prevalence globally. Because of the variety of means used by researchers to assess the disorder in individuals of all ages, the research team concluded that the prevalence range is still a mystery. For example, the ranges cited went from 0.21–57.50 percent in the general population to 50.42–79.25 percent in populations undergoing clinical treatment for an assessed severe case of IGD. Most studies reviewed were conducted in the Republic of Korea, China, and the United States, where IGD rates have been concerning. Across these jurisdictions, mental health experts say that the five most frequently reported symptoms of concern in clients were depression (67 times), internet addiction (54 times), anxiety (48 times), impulsiveness (37 times), and ADHD (24 times).

Case 5. Popi Uses an App to Help Reduce Her Social Media Use

Popi felt that she was spending excessive amounts of time communicating with her high school friends on *Facebook*, particularly via her smartphone. Popi thought to herself, "What do I do now? My school achievement is decreasing rapidly, I feel tired during the day, I'm having difficulty concentrating at school, and I'm not able to sleep through the night!"

Popi told her friend Joan, "I'm really concerned I'm overdoing my 'connect' with our buddies on *Facebook* at all hours of the day and night, but I don't want to miss out on any of their news, and this is the perfect way for me to stay in the know!"

Joan suggested, "Popi, why not just delete the *Facebook* app from your phone if you're that worried? Go on the platform *only* when you're on your computer."

Popi replied, "That would kill me! No, I think I'll download the *Freedom* app on my smartphone instead. I looked it up online and according to its tagline, the app would block sites deemed to be problematic for me—keeping me off them for *just* eight hours at a time. Maybe bedtime would be the perfect eight-hour time slot."

Joan then asked, "Okay, that seems like a doable option for you, but how popular is it?"

Popi responded, "Thought you'd never ask! I was really impressed when I saw that *Freedom's* tagline boasted it 'is used by over 1,000,000 people to reclaim their focus and productivity and to experience the freedom to do what matters most.'"

Joan then asked, "Okay, that's impressive, but what made you become concerned that social media platforms like *Facebook* are bad for your health and well-being and that their usage should be moderated?"

Popi then blurted out,

My school grades are tanking, I can't concentrate at school, and I can't get to sleep or stay asleep at night. Mom and Dad would be really mad if they knew this. Plus, I heard at school that social media platforms are actually engineered to keep us users 'hooked' or even become addicted! Plus, my teacher said that *Facebook* and *X* use our personal information that we supply when we sign up to the site for other profit-making purposes, such as sending us targeted ads geared to our Likes. Look, Joan, I'm convinced I can turn things around for the better by downloading *Freedom*. After all, I read that *Freedom's* purpose is to "give you back your control."

Joan then asked, "Okay, so what if this is just false advertising and this app doesn't help you regain your focus and your marks at school. Then what will you do?"

"Good question," Popi said. "Then I would seriously consider seeking assistance from our school's mental health counselor to help me find other ways to regain control."

Analysis

Popi is smart to try to control her social media platform over-use before mental and physical health issues intensify, possibly leading to an online addiction. She currently admits that her well-being is being adversely impacted by her social media over-use, given that her school productivity is deteriorating as well as her sleep. Though she hasn't openly admitted it, she likely checks her smartphone throughout the night for text messages and emails from friends.

There are a number of options Popi has at this recognized stage of over-use. For starters, Popi should *not* take her smartphone into her bedroom at night, so she can eliminate blue light transmission and get a more restful and refueling night's sleep. Her intention to install an app like *Freedom*—or one of the many other downloadable apps, software add-ons, or program extensions available to help her regain her focus—is also a smart move.

Also, there are a number of built-in features on her smartphone meant to help curb screen time. She may want to use the grayscale functionality to save her phone's battery power and to make attention-getting bright app icons less obvious. She could also disable "notifications" to alleviate attention-demanding alerts while at school or during the night. Popi might also try routinely doing a weekend "digital detox" with her buddies to take a break from their excessive technology use, even for a short period of time. If these readily-available and inexpensive "self-help" options do not reduce Popi's concerning smartphone over-use, she would be wise to make an appointment with her school's mental health counselor to share her concerns and to get some other intervention options for regaining control over her life, including planning more land-based connections with friends to catch up with their news.

For years now, mental health experts (as suggested by Popi's teacher) have articulated that the algorithms employed by social media platforms are intended to persuade young people to be "fully engaged" in the social networking site, encouraging them to return for more novel activities and content—thus reinforcing their habitual use, if not addiction. Also known in the mental health literature as "deliberate persuasive design," Dr. Jeffrey Fogg of Stanford University's Behavior Design lab argues that these practices—no matter how strongly argued as being ethical by social media platforms to "enhance the user experience," clearly violate ethical guidelines precluding deception and coercion.

A similar argument was earlier advanced by former Google design ethicist Tristan Harris, founder of the Center for Human Technology, when he maintained that much of the technology used today on social networking sites operate like a slot machine in casinos. So whether the company is *Facebook* or *Twitter* (now *X*), when designing addictive technology, individuals employed by these companies work on eliciting a particular social response from online users. Thus, designers purposely model a target behavior, or attitude, and enforce it by rewarding users with positive feedback and social support in the users' times of greatest psychological need—through social media notifications of Likes, retweets, and comments.

Is this practice ethical? Probably not, but it keeps online users like Popi coming back for more. She may think her return to *Facebook* is motivated simply by her fear of missing out on her friends' activities, but there is likely much more at play here.

Glossary

Anxiety: An unpleasant emotional experience varying in degree from mild unease to intense dread associated with the anticipation of impending or future disaster. The two main types are recurrent panic attacks and generalized anxiety disorder. Panic attacks occur unexpectedly and can arise in almost any high-stress situation—such that an individual experiences impending doom and outward signs of distress like breathlessness, dizziness, and tingling in the hands or feet. Generalized anxiety disorder is characterized as unrealistic or excessive worry over time and in a number of settings.

Cognitive behavioral therapy (CBT): An effective psychotherapy treatment for compulsive disorders, such as pathological gambling, substance abuse, recurrent panic attacks, and online addiction. Clients are taught not only to monitor their thoughts to identify provoking addictive feelings and actions but to hone new coping skills to prevent relapses.

Copyright Infringement: The act of violating the exclusive rights of a copyright owner by copying, performing, or distributing a work without the owner's permission or by creating the work of one's own that derives from the copyrighted work and for which no credit is given.

Cyberbullying: Bullying someone using electronic communication tools with an intent to cause psychological harm and distress in another online user by issuing unwanted, obnoxious acts by capitalizing on a power imbalance.

Cyberstalking: Using harassing, threatening, or extorting behaviors repeatedly in the virtual space to gain psychological control over a targeted individual by imparting an extreme sense of fear in the target—perhaps even threatening him or her with death or extortion.

Depression: As a mood, it is part of the normal range of experience, usually developing in response to some frustration in life. As a syndrome, it consists of a depressive mood, together with other outward signs of distress like weight loss or an inability to concentrate. As a clinical illness, it involves both the syndrome of depression and the notion that the state is not transitory but is associated with significant functional impairment.

Digital Detox: A periodic disconnect from social or online media to reduce one's stress levels and to focus on maintaining or regaining "mindful" relationships with other individuals in the land-based world—as well as with oneself.

Digital Detox Manifesto: The belief that technology should serve as tools to connect individuals instead of distracting, disturbing, or disrupting them. These technologies should be created mindfully and ethically by the tech industry for the benefit of users rather than to put them in harm's way to make a profit. Simply put, the relationship that grows between the tech creators and the end-users should be truly symbiotic and honest rather than profit-driven.

Hacking: Also known as "cracking," when a perpetrator or set thereof gains illegal access to a network by exploiting gaps in the system's programs (i.e., the operating systems, the drivers, or the communications protocols) and/or by using social engineering.

Social Engineering: A manipulative ploy used by malinclined hackers to create a sense of fear, urgency, or trust in some targeted employee to exploit his or her human error to illegally gain access to a network to steal personally identifiable information (PII) of employees/ clients or to steal proprietary company data.

Directory of Resources

This directory has been compiled to give you additional book and website resources to consult regarding the many important healthy technology use topics covered in this book.

Books

Holt, T.J., & Schell, B.H. (2013). *Contemporary world issues: Hackers and hacking*. Santa Barbara, CA: ABC-CLIO. Discusses topics like the growth and adoption of the internet by mainstream users, how unauthorized network access is gained by the bad actors, and North American laws for sanctioning criminals causing harms to online users.

Kulesza, J. (2012). *International internet law*. Abingdon: Routledge. Looks at international legal issues related to internet governance—including copyright protection, cyberterrorism, identity theft, and fake internet websites—by focusing on China, the United States, the European Union, and Singapore.

Miller, W.R., & Rollnick, S. (2013). *Motivational interviewing: Helping people change*. New York: Guilford Press. Provides a detailed look at how this form of psychotherapy can be used by mental health experts to help online addicted users to recover.

Mitnick, K.D., & Simon, W.L. (2003). *The art of deception: Controlling the human element of security*. New York: John Wiley and Sons, Inc. Kevin Mitnick, likely the world's most infamous hacker sent to US federal prison for a number of years for his costly hacking exploits, discusses the human element of successful network hacks known as "Social Engineering." He explains in this intriguing book why all the firewalls and encryption protocols available on the market cannot stop a tech-savvy hacker who is also very skilled in social engineering from exploiting a network.

Schell, B.H. (2016). *Online health and safety: From cyberbullying to internet addiction*. Santa Barbara, CA: Greenwood. Gives a detailed look at online issues such as internet and gaming addiction, cyberbullying, cyberextortion, identity theft, internet fraud, copyright infringement, and obscene and offensive online content.

Schell, B.H. (2022). *Digital detox: Why taking a break from technology can improve your well-being*. Santa Barbara, CA: Greenwood. Provides a detailed look at the types of internet addictions, ways to measure and treat them, the evolution of the digital detox countermovement, the effectiveness of digital detox holidays and tourism, the Digital Detox Company's focus on Camp Grounded, and fighting technology with technology to improve one's well-being.

Sinacore, A.L., & Ginsberg, F. (2015*). Canadian counselling and counselling psychology in the 21st century.* Montreal and Kingston: McGill-Queen's University Press. Looks at how mental health practitioners view changing trends regarding counseling psychology in the internet age, including the need for online counseling.

Singer, A. (2010). *Alexis: My true story of being seduced by an online predator (louder than words).* Deerfield Beach, FL: Health Communications. Presents a true story about a high school teen lured online by an older man and convinced to put embarrassing personal things of herself on the internet—that she later very much regretted.

Van Der Linden, S. (2023). *Foolproof: Why misinformation infects our minds and how to build immunity.* New York: W.W. Norton. Discusses from a misinformation expert's point of view why our human brains are vulnerable to misinformation and fake news, how and why it spreads so quickly in social media, and strategies we can use to make ourselves more immune from falling prey to it.

Young, K.S. (1998). *Caught in the Net: How to recognize the signs of internet addiction and a winning strategy for recovery.* New York: John Wiley & Sons. Presents from a psychological point of view the "red flags" of internet addiction and provides some very useful steps to help online users heal from it.

Websites

BetterHelp: https://www.betterhelp.com
Offers a "professional therapy made simple" venue to help online users gain access to over 34,000 licensed and experienced mental health counselors in various locations. The therapy delivery is conducted 100 percent online, with a matching of therapist to user made after the user completes an online questionnaire provided on the web site.

Digital Detox: https://www.digitaldetox.com
Details the Digital Detox Company's mission, gives details on upcoming digital detox experiences like Camp Grounded, and provides online users with their own digital awareness scores.

HealthyPlace: https://www.healthyplace.com
Offers psychological tests, a bookstore, mental health videos, blogs, and pointers on how to locate qualified professionals for online users concerned about their well-being.

Internet & Tech Addicts Anonymous: https://netaddictionanon.com

Details a twelve-step fellowship program for addicted online users, created by The
    Internet and Tech Addicts Anonymous (ITAA) group, to bring hope, resources, and
    personal support to individuals confronting online addiction.

iSAFE: www.isafe.org

Details the nonprofit foundation's aims to protect young online users by incorporating
    specially designed classroom curricula with community outreach to empower
    students, their teachers, their parents, and law enforcement to help educate youth
    about staying safe in the online space.

Motion Picture Association: "Watch It Legally" https://www.motionpictures.org/
    watch-it-legally/

Details how the Motion Picture Association (MPA), intending to curb illegal
    downloading and streaming from piracy websites, views the importance of
    copyright protection for creators and their distributors and provides an entertaining
    hub for interviews and stories from behind the scenes—focusing on how consumers'
    favorite movies and TV shows are created.

Net Addiction: http://www.Netaddiction.com

Provides a valuable educational resource for online users to prevent or recover from
    internet addiction by including a series of articles, books, and self-assessment tools
    to help technology users to determine if they have an internet addiction problem for
    which they should seek treatment.

Index

About the Author

Bernadette H. Schell is a well-published professor in the human-computer interaction domain. She is a Professor Emerita in the Faculty of Management at Laurentian University and an Adjunct Professor in the Graduate Faculty of Business and IT at Ontario Tech University, both in Ontario, Canada. She has authored numerous books, including *The Internet and Society*; *Hackers and Hacking*; *Internet Censorship*; and *Digital Detox*—many in Bloomsbury's Contemporary World Issues series. She is coauthor of *Hacking and Technology-Driven Crime: Social Dynamics and Implications* with Dr. Thomas J. Holt at Michigan State University and has written a broad range of journal articles dealing with business and cybercrime.